REVERSING
HUMAN AGING

R E V E R S I N G
HUMAN AGING

MICHAEL FOSSEL, PH.D., M.D.

WILLIAM MORROW AND COMPANY, INC.

New York

It is the policy of William Morrow and Company, Inc., and its imprints and affiliates, recognizing the importance of preserving what has been written, to print the books we publish on acid-free paper, and we exert our best efforts to that end.

Library of Congress Cataloging-in-Publication Data

Fossel, Michael.
    Reversing human aging / Michael Fossel.
        p.   cm.
    Includes bibliographical references and index.
    ISBN 0-688-14324-5
    1. Longevity—Popular works.   I. Title.
QP85.F675   1996
612.6'8—dc20   95-36636
                                                                          CIP

Printed in the United States of America

First Edition

1   2   3   4   5   6   7   8   9   10

BOOK DESIGN BY BONNI LEON-BERMAN

To the truth, no matter how unexpected it may yet be

ACKNOWLEDGMENTS

For their comments, their thoughts, and their thoughtfulness: Jon, Dot, Peter, Les, Scott, Dennis Kolenda, Dwayne Banks, Larry Howard, Eric Ericksen, Aziz Sachedina, Tom Toeller-Novak, Albert Lewis, Daishin Morgan, Karl Scheibe, and Bob Arking. Judges, doctors, rabbis, professors, editors, pastors, lawyers, CEOs, businessmen, scientists, abbots, ethicists, and friends: Thank you. For their undeserved help and their dedication to finding answers to the problems of aging: above all, the special and anonymous crowd out to do in Custer with their BHAGs: Good luck and thank you.

For letting me use the computer when mine died, thanks to VRSH, especially the LSS crew: I owe you.

For being five years old and trying to push me into the swimming pool, my love and hope to Rachel: May she grow young enough to have five-year-olds of her own.

Special thanks to L. Long and RAH.

To the scientists working on aging and disease: The work is theirs, the hopes are ours, the mistakes are mine alone; especially CBH who did much of the work, encouraged the book and the thought, and who is my friend. (PS: I'll win the bet in a hundred years.)

To Laura, who kept the most important people in line and kept a grip.

To Len Hayflick, for finding the truth and telling others.

To Peter Smit, who is part of it; Henry Morrison, who let me tell it; and John Harney, who recognized it.

Joy, Gioia, Ma Joyeuse, more than anyone else, who is, who believed, and whom I love.

To Zan and Lily, who needed just one more thing in the library.

And especially to Virginia Among the Forget-me-nots: *We never will.*

CONTENTS

CONTENTS

INTRODUCTION

THIS BOOK STEMS FROM THE RESEARCH OF MANY OTHER SCIENTISTS, who deserve the credit, as I do not. Those doing the work focus on cells and disease. Most of these researchers feel that discussions about extending longevity beyond its current limits are premature. They are correct. But all of us are not researchers, and it is the implications of their research, and the possibilities that those implications suggest, that make this book both exciting and necessary. While each of them deserves the credit, not one of them is to blame for any interpretation I have made of their work. This book is a presentation of my opinion alone.

Most scientists, those represented in this book among them, work hard to discern fact from speculation, and data from interpretation. Although the first half of this book describes the state of the art in the biology of aging, the second half expresses what I believe is likely to happen, not what I know will happen. It is important that I make the distinction.

Extrapolation and the discussion of possibilities are critical to all of us individually and as a race. The ability to foresee, even dimly and erroneously, the implications of what we have discovered often tempers the results, allowing us to guide our future into more humane channels, finding grace and enlightenment where we might otherwise have fallen into darker paths.

But extrapolation is chancy at best. The errors, the overly bold simplifications, the misunderstandings, all these are my mistakes alone. They are not due to the intemperate overreaching of the thoughtful people who have done the real work. I hope that those of you, scientists and others, who read this book and find apt reason to criticize will lay these errors at my door only. Although all the credit lies with those who are doing the work, the extrapolations and, perhaps at times, unreasonable conclusions that I have drawn from their work are my fault and my own doing.

The facts belong to those who have dedicated their lives to under-standing and to helping; the possibilities belong to all of us. In dis-cussing aging, or any other area of science, we stand between two extremes: certainty and ignorance. Neither extreme is appropriate. Cer-tainty is insupportable; how can we know anything with certainty? Professed ignorance is always a supportable stance, but it is impractical and valueless. Finding an appropriate middle ground involves compro-mises: personal, philosophical, and professional. Were this a book for scientists alone, I would stand closer to ignorance and the book would be more acceptable to them. It is not such a book. Much of it will be criticized harshly. That criticism is justified: I have gone beyond my facts. I have done so knowingly; perhaps that is the greater fault.

I have elected to tempt fate and encourage critics by leaning further toward certainty than many will find acceptable. It was my choice and I will live with it. Perhaps you suspect that I look forward to the criticism. I do not. But I do look forward to finding out what the truth is, and I look forward to the future. The future may not be at hand, but it is not far off.

LIFE

THE HORIZON

Only the gods live forever ...
but as for us men, our days are numbered,
our occupations are a breath of wind.

—*The Epic of Gilgamesh*, 3000 B.C.

THIS BOOK IS a promise and a warning. It is a promise of a time when we will live longer and much healthier lives—of one hundred, two hundred, possibly five hundred years. It is also a warning of what could happen when we do. It tells little about diet, very little about coping with aging, and nothing about whether one should choose to age or not. What it says is that we will have a choice.

We will be able to prevent, even reverse, aging within two decades. At the same time, and as part of the same process, we will also cure most of the diseases that now frighten and destroy us. Cancer, a disease in which malignant cells refuse to age, will be among the first to go. Instead of being a source of terror and tragedy, it will become a bad memory, an inconvenience. Diseases that we think of as part of growing old could soon disappear. By profoundly increasing our "health span," we will also increase the human life span. When we do, we will change human society in ways we will applaud, ways we will regret, and ways we cannot foresee. This book is the story of how we are conquering aging and of what the consequences will be. It is the story of our hopes and our fears, and of change that will soon shake our world. We are about to change history forever.

THE HOUSE OF AGING

No house should ever be on any hill or on anything. It should be of the hill, belonging to it, so hill and house could live together each the happier for the other.

—FRANK LLOYD WRIGHT

Is reversing human aging hypothetical? No. The work is unfinished, but not hypothetical.

If I build a house, when does it change from a dream to a home? For years it is only a wish. Then, for a time, it lives only as a clumsy set of napkin sketches, rumpled and confused, but hopeful. The dream firms, plans are drawn and changed; a bank signs a loan, a builder is contracted, a bulldozer snorts and twists across the site; a hole is dug, a foundation poured, the frame rises. Is the house now still a dream or is it real?

This is the stage at which we tell our story. The framing is in place, the roof is on, the walls are rising. The house is not yet ready to live in, but it soon will be. Is it hypothetical? No, only unfinished.

This particular house began with a man named Leonard Hayflick. He marked the site where today the house rises. Thirty-five years ago, as a young researcher in Philadelphia, Hayflick found that all the normal body cells he grew eventually died no matter what he did. Len Hayflick was annoyed and chagrined. The prevailing and unchallenged belief of that day, a fact that everyone knew, was that individual cells—with care—lived forever in the laboratory. Yet Hayflick could not make them survive. No matter how many times he tried, no matter what he did, unless he added new cells, Hayflick watched his normal cells divide a set number of times and then stop. Always they stopped. Anxious, but certain of his results, he published a series of papers that brought him criticism and ridicule . . . and finally fame. Hayflick's papers became classics, for they describe the hill on which the house of aging now rises. Of all that we know about aging, Hayflick's work, high and commanding, stands out above the landscape.

For three decades the hill stood vacant. Then in 1990, a handful of scientists, including Cal Harley at McMaster University in Canada and Bruce Futcher and Carol Greider at Cold Spring Harbor Laboratory in New York, began to build on it. It was Hayflick who said that all our cells must age and die; it was this new generation who found the clock that times their death. Their work had begun in the mid-seventies and their sketches became the blueprints of the house by 1990. Those who understood the plans helped them build and the house began to rise. It stands now, more than half built, no longer a dream, but not yet finished.

There are two milestones in the story of aging: Len Hayflick's proof that cells age, and the more recent discovery that they don't have to. Cells have chromosomal "clocks" that determine their life spans. A cell dies when its clock runs down. Cancer cells, on the other hand, continually reset their clocks, allowing themselves to divide forever. If we reset the clock of a normal cell, it lives anew; if we stop the clock of a cancer cell, it dies. When we can set the clocks, your cells need not age and cancer can be cured.

Although you are far more than a collection of separate cells whose clocks can be reset, your body need not age as it does today. The biological technology for achieving this, the unfinished part of the house, is still in progress. In this book, we will look over the blueprints and drawings of the house, follow its construction, and see which parts are ready for us now and which parts are still unfinished.

We will explore the question of what we can cure and what still lies beyond our ability. Alzheimer's and heart disease, for example, will become trivial and rare. Cancer will give way completely. But health and long life are not the whole story.

When the house is finished, we will live in it. Some will complain: The house is too new, the style unfamiliar, the rooms not what they wanted. Most of us, however, will be happy to be in from the cold, out of the rain, and safe from the wind. Most of us will find a home that we will come to love and be grateful for.

Today it is a matter of finishing the work. In ten years, perhaps twenty, it may be completed, with only the furniture lacking.

THE SPIRIT AND THE DUST

Death is a dialog between
The spirit and the dust.
"Dissolve," says death. The spirit, "Sir,
I have another trust."

—EMILY DICKINSON

Life is a trust. It is a trust that you hold not only for yourself, but for those you love, and for all living things. There is a joy, an élan, a spirit to life that is far more important than its duration. That spirit is so closely akin to our health that we might better wish to extend our health span than our life span. Watching those we love sicken and fail, we would wish them longer health over longer life. The enemy is loss and suffering, fear and tragedy. Many of us, therefore, are dedicated to the task of increasing not just a life span, but the quality of life. We wish to add joy and spirit, not just years.

Death is something none of us can avoid, and yet we do not fear death so much as we cherish life. It is more than simply life that we cherish; it is *healthy* life. We value the things that define life for us, and that make it worth living: the joy, the excitement, the warmth, the love of those we share it with.

In the last half of the twentieth century, medical advances have kept us alive longer than ever before, but often only by definition. The distinction between mere life and *quality of life* has become profound. We are now able to prolong life without definable limits, but we have done so without any discernible gain. The ethical and financial costs are increasingly painful and troubling.

We prolong mere life and forget that mind and soul must fill it. Instead, our bodies are pushed along by a weary and uncaring attention to a vacant shell. All of this to gain nothing: neither time with friends, nor moments of reflection, nor the excitement of being alive and well, nor the small pleasures that warm us, making us deeper and more human.

Fountains of youth have existed in legends from time immemorial, but have never been more than that: mere legends. History has revealed them to be fantasy: From Gilgamesh to Ponce de León, we have conjured up a cavalcade of groundless wishes and dashed hopes.

Yet history is also made from dreams. Fiction turns to reality, flights of fancy to flights around the world. Smallpox has disappeared; we are blasé as we fly across continents; we watch the earthrise from the moon; computers talk to us and even begin to listen to us, making us wonder if we ourselves could ever learn that skill.

How have we moved from dreams to history? Has it been a sudden and unpredictable shift, a random unfolding of surprises, or has it been an evolution? Why do we make history when we do? We can only weave history from dreams when the threads lie ready in our hands. Those threads are simple ones: knowledge and ability slowly grown from hard work. Unexpectedly, seemingly by a revolution, the threads become a fabric. Engines and airflow become jetliners, little pieces of knowledge join and become a new creation.

You may be offered an opportunity to become twenty again—and remain so—for a far longer time than you have yet lived. You would feel and move and be as healthy as you once were, although some things would not be reversed. Therefore, care well for your teeth—you will not get a third set. Alzheimer's disease may be prevented—not reversed. Heart disease may become rare, but the damage done by heart attacks will not be undone. Menopause may come at the same age as it always has, no matter that you look half that age. Some things, once broken, cannot be repaired; some will occur regardless.

Some things are free; many are not. What will be the costs of turning back our clocks? They will be few—not none, but few. As we will see, the physical costs are likely to be small and trivial compared with other costs—and with the potential gain. What about financial costs? What of social or ethical costs? These will be the greater concerns.

The financial cost will be small if by that we mean only the cost of the treatment. A far greater and more unpredictable cost is that of the change that will sweep us up as our society alters forever. Think of how much depends on the knowledge that we age as we do, that we sicken as we age, and that we die when we do. These have been well-founded assumptions in our lives: How could it be otherwise?

Yet soon it will be. Soon it will all change, for better, for worse, for the unknown. Jobs, investments, laws, governments, social roles, all will shift. The threads that run through our lives will be woven in new and, in some cases, frightening ways before we can learn to accept our longer, healthier life spans and be at ease with who we will soon become.

The change will be gradual at first. Books like this one, articles, interviews, editorials; discussions on television news and talk shows: These will be the first forums, the places where the early tremors will be felt.

As we come to accept the fact that aging can be altered, our lives will change, even before aging is treatable. Your outlook, once confined to decades, will move outward into hesitant centuries. Do you enjoy your job? Do you hate it? Do you look forward to retirement as a time of rest, or resent it as forced idleness? What would you do with an extra century of health and youth? You will not be alone in asking a thousand such questions. The answers, once only fantasy, will now change what you do and how you live. The answers will change us all.

The change will accelerate. Subtle, but pervasive, change will be everywhere. Society will shift and waver. You will quit your job; she will go back to school; he will spend his pension. You will discover that your insurance company is bankrupt and you are out of work; he will discover that sports equipment and real estate are booming; she will discover that her family has changed pleasantly in some ways, disturbingly in others.

Through it all will run a new hope—fueled by newfound health and the excitement of renewed youth and dreams. The ability to do many new things, and the time to finish them, will become reality in the next few decades.

As you might suspect, medical care will alter radically as some diseases, once common, become rare, while others, now unknown, become routine. The difficult question of national health care, now a bone of contention, will change its focus in unpredictable ways. Will the emphasis be on the promotion of ever greater health, with the cost falling as we become younger and healthier? Or will the opposite occur?

Some financial wizards will be gleeful, seeing their own health and prospects improve. Others will develop ulcers as they lose faith in what little they knew—or thought they did—about our economy and the financial markets. Some pension managers will see their jobs changing and new opportunities rising everywhere, while others fight for new regulations, new contracts, and new laws to hold back their losses. Social Security as it exists today will disappear or become unrecognizable. En route, it will become the battleground of angry politicians, loudly debating the legal and ethical questions it will pose anew. Do we scrap Social Security or sculpt it afresh with the chisels of law and finance?

The change will hurt at times and at other times give us hope. Some who first advocated long and healthy lives will reconsider, wondering if they were not better off with known diseases and a short but predictable life. Most of us might mourn the loss of a society we thought we knew and perhaps understood, but will still think it a fair trade for health and boundless time to live. Some of us will eagerly embrace the opportunities and the excitement of the new, accepting of—or oblivious to—the dangers of change. A few will decline longer, healthier lives, for diverse reasons—some religious, some psychological, some unclear and inexpressible. But most will welcome long life, even at the cost of temporary social upheaval and uncertainty.

Why is this happening in our time? Part of the delay has been due to our inability to open our eyes to new possibilities. Believing that flight was impossible, we lacked airplanes; believing many diseases incurable, we did not seek a cure. Our acceptance of the limits of our lives was deeper yet: Aging was not a disease to us, but a fact of life. And so it would have remained, but for those who questioned that fact and tried to change it.

In this century we have finally begun to understand enough about ourselves to extend our own lives. Developments in biochemistry, genetics, medicine, and a dozen other fields, and improvements in microscopes, antibodies, gene sequencing, and two hundred other techniques have all contributed.

For most of this century, our knowledge of aging was a puzzle with hundreds of pieces missing spread out on the table before us. Every year brought new pieces to the table; every year we fit a few more of them together. Most researchers have concentrated on finding the missing pieces, working hard at understanding the few hard-won facts we could wrestle from our aging bodies. A few concentrated on putting the whole puzzle together. It was a thankless, seemingly impossible task; the pieces were well cut, the colors crisp, the patterns well defined, yet they did not make a cohesive picture. Here there were bits of a still life, there of a raucous party; here was part of a church in autumn, there a few spring apple blossoms. Throughout, there was no theme, no single clue as to how these pieces fit together. There was no way of joining them into one puzzle—until the past few years.

In the late 1980s, hints began to appear about the overall picture. In the past few years, the edge pieces that bound the puzzle have finally come together. Today we see a single picture and discover to our vast surprise that all our pieces, once disparate and disjointed, relate to a single theme.

The theme is, as Emily Dickinson said, a dialogue between the spirit and the dust. To understand the dialogue, we will need to know the players and what they are saying to us. We need to understand a bit about life and immortality, about the dust and the spirit. Let us begin with the first two of these: life and immortality.

LIFE AND IMMORTALITY

…Nothing in his life
Became him like the leaving it; he died
As one that had been studied in his death,
To throw away the dearest thing he ow'd,
As 'twere a careless trifle.

—*MACBETH, I.IV*

Immortality is everywhere. There has been life on this planet for three and a half billion years, and it will continue when you and I are gone. The cell line that you inherited from your parents can be traced back to our planet's dawn, when Earth lay almost barren of life. The process of life is immortal, but the individual is not. Although we may increase our life span by hundreds of years, death remains inevitable. All the cells in our bodies are mortal; we are immortal only in looking backward at whence we have come. No matter how we might alter our genes, no matter how healthy we are, no matter how young we become, we will still be mortal.

Although we cannot escape mortality, we can avoid aging. Aging is a process that now occurs in almost all of our cells. The exception is our germ cells, our sperm or ova. Curiously enough, those cells don't age as the rest do. They haven't aged since life began; they never will.

Germ cells have carried genes from generation to generation until they formed you. We can follow their line backward through your parents, your grandparents, your furthest ancestors, back to the beginnings of life. This is the small part of you that has so far actually *been* immortal.

Along the way, there has been change, of course. As time passed, over billions of years, the genes in your germ cell line have been altered by mutation and exchange. The genes have changed, but the line of inheritance continued. Genes were lost and new ones replaced them, but the line remained immortal. It is a curious will-o'-the-wisp immortality.

Nonetheless, your genes have a share in this immortality. They are perpetuated in your children, in your children's children, echoing into future generations until, perhaps, your line dies out and becomes extinct. Yet, you are far more than a carrier of genes. You are a knowing, thinking being, capable of self-awareness, self-direction, and even self-destruction. Most likely, you treasure your life, even though it is short, particularly when compared with your billion-year-old genes.

Why this remarkable contrast? If the thread of life is immortal, why are our lives so short? The answer to this question is initially quite straightforward, but as we will later see, the full answer holds the key to both cancer and aging. Your body, excepting your germ cells, is made up of cells that age and die, known as somatic cells. Just as your somatic cells die, so will you: if not of infection, then of heart disease, cancer, stroke, or some other malady. And if not of one of these, then of trauma or the next astronomical disaster that catapults our species into extinction as happened to the dinosaurs sixty-five million years ago.

But what about aging? Is aging, like death, inevitable? Again, the answer is straightforward. Unlike death, aging *can* be avoided. It can even be reversed. We already know that some of our cells can avoid aging. Germ cells die but they do not age.[1] They are unique among all of the trillions of other cells that make up the human body. How can these cells, with the same genes, the same dangers, the same membranes, and the same metabolic wastes remain unaffected by all the forces that age other cells?

There are master clocks that run down in our somatic cells and that can be reset. To understand how they work, we first need to understand our own bodies a bit better. What happens to our genes and to our cells that finally destroys us as we age?

Genes are the blueprints for the cell's activities. These activities have a grand purpose: to support our remarkably complex organisms in the face of an environment that tends to tear us apart and wear us down. Systems fall apart, order unravels into chaos: This tendency toward disruption is called entropy.

In life, entropy—the second law of thermodynamics—operates with a vengeance. Entropy is in a constant war with biological forces that try to maintain a well-controlled, "homeostatic" environment for the cell. Homeostasis is the tendency for a biological system to keep things steady and unchanged. When you become dehydrated, you drink; when you are cold, you shiver; when your blood sugar falls, you eat. More important, when a cell runs out of a molecule, it produces more; when it has too many, it breaks down the surplus or pumps out the excess; for every imbalance, the cell reacts. The defensive homeostatic forces are well-balanced overall, yet ultimately homeostasis fails, you age, and finally you die.

These two forces—entropy and homeostasis—are not the only two players in the biological balance, however. There is a third set of players—the clocks that tell time in every cell in your body. They are the central theme of this book. Stop them, and you stop the aging process; turn them back and you actually turn back aging. We will first meet the clocks in cell cultures, where they limit cells to a finite number of divisions called, appropriately enough, the Hayflick limit. The cell stops dividing and finally dies despite all attempts to optimize its environment. This is the first clue in our search for an understanding of aging.

But what is aging?

Can it be merely "wear and tear"? Is it simply a surrender to unavoidable damage or merely a loss of immune function? Is it suffocation in metabolic waste or just leaking membranes? Or is it the result of actively turning off your defenses as some deep cellular clock ticks down to a final stop?

What characteristics does the clock have, where is it, and how will we know it when we find it? These are the questions that we must address and ultimately answer in order to alter and reverse aging. These are the questions that occupy our first few chapters.

To begin, let us look at what aging acts upon. Let us look more closely at your cells, the finely wrought parts of your body, and the genes that hold the designs you were made from.

CELLS BY MICHELANGELO

Lump the whole thing!
Say that the Creator made Italy from designs by Michael
    Angelo!

—MARK TWAIN, *THE INNOCENTS ABROAD*

Your body is made up of cells. While not large, you are extraordinarily crowded. An accurate count of all the cells has never been made, and perhaps never will be, but there are well in excess of a trillion of them—perhaps a 100 trillion—that lump themselves into the intricate design that is you.[2] Michelangelo could never have done as well.

Each individual cell is different. They differ in location, in function, and in appearance. Some, like your liver cells, are almost identical, yet they are still distinct in subtle ways. There are innumerable different kinds of cells: liver cells, brain cells, lung cells, muscle cells, and so on. All differ, not only in their anatomy, but in how they act. Each individual cell has its own biochemical fingerprint and no two are exact duplicates.

It is as though your cells were each at the tips of the twigs of a gigantic, almost infinitely branched tree, each branch marking the point where two cells divided and grew their separate ways. Some, like liver cells, are closely related, their twigs touching, expressing almost the same interpretation of their common genes. Some, like skin cells and blood cells, are far apart, as though on opposite sides of the tree, sharing only the common trunk. The trunk is the fertilized egg, the joined sperm and ovum that divided and branched into different cells.

Sperm and ovum met, shared their genes, compared notes, and began dividing. Even from those first few divisions, there were differences as branches split and then split again. Although most of the trunk was bound upward to create all of the cells of your body—the somatic cells—a few quite special cells branched off as the trunk left the ground.

Those few cells are the germ cells, they alone do not age. They have a special purpose, to form new sperm in males and eggs in females. They are separated anatomically from your somatic cells, coddled and protected, and remain separate genetically. No matter what might happen to your somatic genes, the germ cell genes will be a legacy for your children. They are the future and they represent your past.

Every branch of the tree, every cell, has a reference library from the past: the gene collection. Half of the books were donated by your mother, half by your father. All of the books are shelved together in a common library and are found in nearly every cell. The library is the same in all cells, germ or somatic.

The library tells the cell what to become and how it should differ from others; as the cells divide, one may become a developing nerve cell, another a developing blood cell. At every division, the positions of the cells in the embryo, along with the blueprints themselves, determine what each cell will be. Throughout life, the library also directs the day-to-day housekeeping chores of the cell, maintaining and repairing it continuously. Both of the library's functions, development and maintenance, play a role in our understanding of aging. But first, we need an understanding of the cell's library.

Like any library, the cell's has books, sentences, words, and letters. The books in this library are the chromosomes, long, chained molecules on which are written the genes, which are the sentences. All the chromosomes together make up the library—or genome—of the cell.

And in this fashion, the library embodies the complete collection of all the genes in the cell and every cell has the complete library of genes.

Genome—Library
Chromosome—Book
Gene—Sentence
DNA Base—Letter

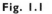

Fig. 1.1

The knowledge written in these books, the gene sentences that are found on each page, create our abilities and define much of our existence. In each sentence lies information we need, not only to construct our bodies as we grow from fetus to adult, but also to reconstruct them minute by minute, as changes occur in the environment or as the molecular pieces of the organism are damaged, broken down, and lost.

This breaking down is natural and even necessary. It occurs both accidentally, as the environment damages molecules within the cells, and intentionally, as the cells take apart and recycle their components. Each of your cells is continuously in flux, even after you become an adult, when there is little or no obvious change. Moment by moment, the molecules and parts of cells are torn down, rebuilt, and refashioned. Your cells constantly refer back to the cellular library, checking the schematic diagrams and instructions printed there that allow you to continuously and accurately remodel and repair yourself. Yet as you age, the recycling slows down, remodeling becomes halfhearted, repair an occasional affair.

How is the knowledge transmitted from your library to the workshops and factories of your cells? The chromosome sentence is a long chain of DNA letters. The information is copied from your DNA onto RNA, much as information is loaded from a computer onto a disk. The RNA disk copy is taken from the library and brought to your factories—your ribosomes—where the RNA disk copy becomes a working blueprint, in turn, to build your proteins.

Proteins are the sole output of your cellular factories. Proteins come in three types: structural proteins, signaling proteins, and enzymes. The structural proteins are the framework of your cells: the girders, concrete, and walls. The signaling proteins are messengers, traveling from one cell to another, informing other cells how they should respond. The enzymes are the machinery: the electrical system, heating, appliances, and tools.

Enzymes are the great magicians of your cells: They change molecules into other molecules, join one molecule to another, build molecules, and tear them apart. Every molecule in the cell is continuously being built up and torn down by your enzymes. The amount of each molecule in a cell is the moment-to-moment product of the simultaneous building up and tearing down of that molecule. This process creates a delicate, wavering balance. Even the enzymes themselves are continuously torn down and rebuilt, just as they tear apart and rebuild other molecules.

Your DNA library is divided into forty-six chromosomes—the "books." Each book has a not-quite-identical twin, forming twenty-three paired volumes. The copy is almost identical, but not exactly; each is a slightly different version of its twin. The organization of each of the twin books—the table of contents, the chapter headings, the placement of material—is identical, but the information differs slightly. You have two separate opinions as to how to do things. One opinion (one of the twin books) is from your father; the other opinion (the other book) is from your mother.

As in any good marriage, the opinions differ somewhat, but disputes are generally settled amicably. And, occasionally, having a second opinion saves your life. That is true of a number of diseases (such as sickle-cell trait) in which one opinion is clearly wrong: The instructions, if followed to the letter, would kill you. Having a second opinion allows the cell to hedge its bets and survive.

As in some, but by no means all, marriages, there are dominant opinions and yielding opinions. In genetics, these are called dominant and recessive genes. Dominance of a gene is unrelated to which parent it came from, and just as in life, being dominant has nothing—or almost nothing—to do with being right.

Being dominant and wrong is a poor combination. If the dominant gene is dangerous enough, the cell dies. If enough other cells express

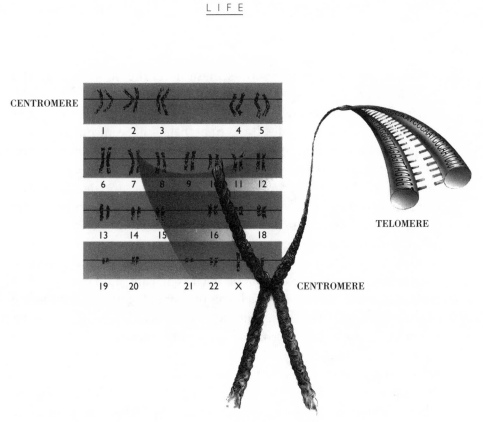

Fig. 1.2

the same fatal gene, the whole body dies. All other things being equal, the fatal gene won't be passed on; however, as things are rarely equal, an enormous variety of genes—including some quite nasty ones—survive in the collective library of our species. Your own library has a collection of genes, some good, some adequate, and a few that you would be embarrassed to admit to.

There are actually two kinds of genetic libraries in each cell: the library of genes in your cell's nucleus and a smaller gene library, containing just one book, in your mitochondria, the power stations of your cells, as it were. The genes in your mitochondria are different and special in several ways, but can be ignored for our purposes. For now, we will focus on the genes in your nuclei.

Most of what we need to know about aging has to do with the larger (150,000 times as large), more important gene library in the nucleus. Each of the forty-six books is a single long molecule of DNA. In a sense, the chromosome is less like a book than a scroll, but since few of us handle scrolls these days, the book analogy is a more apt one.

A typical chromosome book has two "upper arms" and two "lower arms" joined at the middle by a tight belt—the centromere. (Why chromosomes have four arms but no legs has never been clear to anyone.) The four ends—the hands, perhaps?—two on the upper arms and two on the lower arms, of the chromosome are the telomeres. Each set of "arms" (for example, the right upper and lower arms) are formed from a continuous double strand of DNA joined to an identical set of arms (the left upper and lower arms) by the centromere in the middle. So not only do you have pairs of nearly identical books in your genetic library, but each book itself is actually a double strand of DNA, a "double book," in which the two strands form the two facing pages as the book is opened. One side can be read normally; the other is a mirror image, an exact duplicate written backward on the facing page.

Focusing on only one set of pages, the right-hand side, for example, the double strand is an exceedingly long helically twisted strand of DNA running continuously from telomere to telomere. Figure 1.2 shows some of these strands fully wound up, in a quite compact form that is not commonly found in most of your cells, but is seen only at certain times, for example, just before a cell divides. It is as though the cell has squeezed all of its chromosomal library into a few very well-packed boxes in order to move to a new home. During this phase, little if any of the library is actually available for use, having been packed too densely to allow easy access. As we will see, packing important parts of the DNA into boxes, even when you still need it, is part of what happens when you age.

After dividing, the cell unpacks. In most cells, the DNA library is only partially unpacked. The books are partly open, allowing your cells to read some of the information.

The entire library is probably never completely unpacked. Each cell needs only certain "chapters" in each book; the information required depends on the type of cell and on the stage of development. A nerve cell—a neuron—needs information about chemical transmitters, but never opens the chapters on making bone. The bone cell needs to know how to build bone out of phosphorus and calcium, but has no use for the chapters on making muscles. The muscle cell must make muscle proteins, but not antibodies. Each cell type has its own requirements; its own frequently referenced books, well-worn chapters, and bent pages; but every cell has the entire library available, if not in actual use.

In fact, if the whole library were in operation, the cell would be useless or even dangerous to you. Information not absolutely necessary to any particular cell is restricted. The restriction is appropriate, because cells such as cancer cells that access and express genes inappropriately will divide when they shouldn't, produce the wrong molecules, and damage their neighbors. They grow when they shouldn't and where they shouldn't.

Just as cells should express only what is necessary and no more, they must also express no less. Inability to access and express crucial "chapters" and "sentences" from the DNA library results in cell death.

A cell can even be "instructed," by neighboring cells or by hormones from more distant cells, to close down part of its library and die. Once a cell receives its death notice, its "suicide genes" become active. That is probably what happens regularly during menstrual cycles when the uterine lining is sloughed off. You also used this kind of programmed cell death ("apoptosis") prenatally to sculpt yourself, losing the webbing between your toes and fingers, for example.

This is quite different from the more usual cell death ("necrosis") that results from a poor environment. In necrosis, the cells are destroyed by outside forces, not by "suicide." They die because they lack glucose or oxygen, or the temperature is too extreme, or the environment doesn't meet the cell's needs in some other way.

In the case of programmed cell death, on the other hand, the cell has everything it needs to survive except permission. Despite every other metabolic need being met, the cell commits suicide under orders from other cells, because the death is programmed in the genes. The cell is given instructions to die, it only requires that a particular molecular message interacts with a particular set of genes, and death will be the unavoidable outcome.

While your body is forming, your cells have access to parts of the library that they will never need again. Every fetal cell, whether it is a neuron, a skin cell, or any other kind, has separate and temporary requirements for special chapters in your genetic library. As cells divide and differentiate from their siblings, their needs change.

In a mature cell—one that has finally differentiated into a liver cell, bone cell, neuron, etc.—the chromosomes are only partially unwound. Certain chapters in each book can be opened and read; the rest are kept closed. The textbook resemblance of each chromosome to an X no longer pertains. Instead, the chromosome is a long, confusing collection of spaghettilike strands within the cell's nucleus. Portions of each chromosome, the euchromatin, or "true chromatin," are unwound (the unpacked part of the library); while others, the heterochromatin ("other chromatin"), remain tightly wound and unavailable (still in boxes). The heterochromatin and the telomere at the end of each chromosome play key roles in aging. To understand what those roles are, we need to understand the genes themselves a bit better.

If you were to unwind the chromosome completely, you would find a long molecule of DNA composed of only four DNA bases: adenine, guanine, thymine, and cytosine. These bases are usually simply abbreviated and known by their first letters (that is all that will be needed in this book): A, G, T, and C.

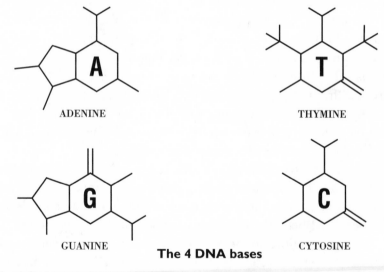

ADENINE

THYMINE

GUANINE

CYTOSINE

The 4 DNA bases

Fig. 1.3

These four bases make up the alphabet in which the sentences in each book in your genetic library are written. A chromosome is a long chain of repetitive DNA bases—for example, ATTAGCCTAGGACC . . .—beginning at one telomere and ending (perhaps 130 million letters later) at the other. This single DNA strand, as just discussed, has a complementary or "negative" strand that attaches to it like a zipper. In the two complementary chains, A is always paired with T; G, with C. So if one strand read ATCG, the other would read TAGC, its "negative" in this sense. The fact that you have two strands allows you to re-create lost pieces on either strand. If one strand is missing a letter, but the other still has a "T," then an "A" must be missing. Having two strands enables you to repair your genes.

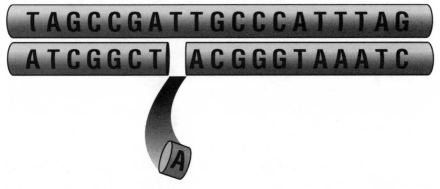

Fig. 1.4

The strands are so long that they are often referred to in groups of thousands of bases, or kilobases, abbreviated kb. Adding together all forty-six of your chromosome books, you have approximately 3 billion letters—3 million kb—in your genome library. Although it might seem useful to refer to chromosomes not in kilobases, but in some even larger unit, kilobase units are a better choice when we talk about individual genes, whose lengths are in this range.

Genes are the sentences in your genetic books; these sentences range from 10 to 200 kb in length—10,000 to 200,000 letters long—each having as many letters as there are words in this book. Any sentence that long needs substantial editing, which is what you do. It is as though in each sentence in the books, there are a variable number of nonsense words (called introns) that need to be ignored before we can understand the meaning and create anything useful. But from the important words (called exons) the editing rules are still only poorly understood.

Your cells don't just make proteins automatically, regardless of whether they are needed or not. As with everything else that your cells do, making proteins is carefully regulated. The growing chain of amino acids that is a new protein has to be started, encouraged to grow longer, stopped when it is finished, and then released. Changes at any of these stages will affect how much protein your cells make: increasing it, slowing it, or even stopping it. "Elongation factors," for example, are critical to helping the protein grow to its full, normal length. These factors are some of the primary control mechanisms as you age. If these elongation factors decrease—which happens as you age—protein production will decrease.

It may seem that the process of going from gene to protein is complex. It is, but knowledge of most of it is unnecessary to understanding the basic process of aging. This introduction represents only the barest, most simplified outline of the process.

Because it is so complex, the process of going from genes to proteins is fraught with opportunities for error and mistranslation of the blueprints. A single misread gene among billions of letters, a tiny mistake in production, or a single wrong amino acid among thousands on a protein may result in an apparently small change in protein function. Yet that small change may have vast consequences for the organism. There are numerous cases in which a single wrong amino acid in the making of a single protein has proved fatal (for instance, sickle-cell disease).

Yet, surprisingly, almost shockingly, both the cells and the entire organism generally survive for several decades of life and even flourish. Your germ cell line has survived for billions of years. You continuously read and translate your library flawlessly as judged by the result: You are alive and generally healthy.

Maintenance of your library and translation from your genes are fragile, almost frighteningly delicate functions on which you balance. But the genes are not alone in maintaining this delicate balance. All of your proteins—in fact all of the molecules in your cells—are continuously created and destroyed. The destruction occurs both intentionally and accidentally. Your cells intentionally destroy and rebuild molecules continuously; nature damages molecules continuously, but does not spontaneously rebuild.

The intentional destruction has a purpose. You carefully regulate the concentration of each kind of molecule and dilute damaged molecules in a pool of newly minted, normal ones. Every protein—for instance, SOD (superoxide dismutase), a common antioxidant protein that is important to the aging process[3]—is continuously created and broken down. Both the creation and breakdown are active processes, and both are actively *regulated* processes. If the cell needs more SOD, it can either increase production or decrease the breakdown. Any change in either production or breakdown will alter the amount of SOD in your cells.

In the same sense, the enzymes responsible for production and degradation of SOD are also regulated. If you want more of the enzymes that produce the protein, you can either create more of *those* enzymes or slow *their* breakdown. The same is true of these enzymes in turn, as well as of the enzymes responsible for breaking down the protein. This tree of regulatory processes can be followed back step by step to the translation from the DNA library itself.

Your cells have dozens of regulatory points to control protein production and destruction. Each level of regulation is also affected by multiple inputs: One regulatory step may be affected most by calcium, another by glucose, a third by hormones, and so forth in endless complexity. Access to the gene is regulated. Certain sentences in the book are off limits unless special conditions occur in the cell. A neuron should not make bone, nor should a bone cell make muscle. The genes in your library are controlled by regulatory genes, which act as the librarians, allowing access to some genes, forbidding access to others.

Regulatory genes prohibit or allow reading of other genes; repressing genes inhibit the translation of their associated genes; activating genes promote the translation of their genes.

The regulatory genes are themselves regulated, although what does so is not obvious. We might—whimsically, but with a loose accuracy—say that they are regulated by everything and anything that comes near the cell. We already understand the general process and—in a few specific cases—understand it quite well.

From inside the cell, the regulatory genes receive feedback from the proteins whose levels they regulate and from the molecules that the proteins affect. Too much product causes the regulator to slow down production; too little causes the regulator to speed it up. From outside the cell, hormones, other messengers (so-called trophic factors), and the environment affect gene regulation. Some hormones—thyroid, retinoids, and steroids of all sorts—affect the regulators directly; others do so indirectly. Messenger molecules from nearby cells dictate whether a cell may divide or how it differentiates—into what type of cell, for example—or even if it should die. Finally, changes in your external environment—temperature, for example—also affect gene expression.

Regulatory genes control other regulatory genes in a cascade of uncertain dimensions. Like a biological Rube Goldberg contraption, gene A activates the translation of gene B, which in turn both activates translation of gene C and represses gene D translation. Gene C represses the expression of gene A (which started the whole intricate process), completing a feedback circuit and thereby shutting itself down again. Truly mind-boggling prospects can be imagined, with endlessly nested regulatory programs.

There are also master genes, major regulators of gene expression. The classic example is the homeobox, a sequence of genes responsible for overall regulation of major portions of fetal development.

All of this regulation is complex and interesting (if you are a biochemist), but where does aging fit into all of this regulation? Aging regulates several key processes, for example protein production and DNA repair. Aging turns them down, forcing your cells to slow down and finally stop. It turns off your defenses, surrendering your cells to "the slings and arrows" of the world. What are these forces that try to destroy you? What are the engines of aging?

CHAPTER 2

THE ENGINES OF AGING

NATURAL SHOCKS

The slings and arrows of outrageous fortune,... the thousand
  natural shocks
That flesh is heir to.

—*HAMLET*, III.i

THE NATURAL SHOCKS that strive to break us down are caused by entropy. These are the forces of disorganization, decay, dissolution: "slings and arrows," wear and tear. But entropy is not the same as aging, or the same as death; it is the force that wears you down, whereas aging is the process that abandons you to entropy. Entropy represents one side of a tug-of-war; the other side is fought by your defenses. If you lose that tug-of-war, you lose your life.

Entropy works at all levels, from your smallest genes to the grossest anatomic level. At the finest level we consider—that of the molecule—

entropy spontaneously alters or breaks down your molecules by means of isomerization, free radicals, cross-linked proteins, DNA damage, protein degradation, decreased turnover, and lipofuscin deposition. At the grossest level—that of your whole body—it includes falls, automobile accidents, gunshots, and the "thousand natural shocks that flesh is heir to."

At any level, entropy would be catastrophic if you couldn't avoid it or repair the damage it causes. At the molecular level, your molecules spontaneously mutate into mirror images of themselves: Like Alice passing through the looking glass, they change into an altered form— inside out, backward, inverted. These "isomers" wouldn't be so bad, except that you can only use one of the two forms: In proteins, the left-handed form is normal;[1] the right-handed form is not.[2] You can't use the right-handed form of proteins and you can even be damaged by them. Even this bias of yours would not be a problem if the isomers, once created in the "correct" form (which is how they are always formed) stayed that way, but of course they don't. They slip from one form to the other without warning or announcement.

Your molecules can also undergo more complex metamorphoses. For instance, the amino acids that make up proteins can bond sideways to one another, "kinking" the protein and making it useless. It happens spontaneously and continuously in all of your cells.

Or, less often, your molecules "racemize," forming hodgepodge collections of different isomers—not only isomers that are left-handed and right-handed, but ones that are twisted and rearranged, using the same pieces but making a different pattern. It is as though you took a word and randomly shuffled the letters; the molecule has the same parts, but they are put together in new ways that your genes never intended and that your body doesn't know how to use. Many of these molecules are almost normal, but some are altered into bizarre and unrecognizable shapes. What was once a useful molecule is suddenly a nuisance. It not only doesn't work, but it takes additional trouble to repair. This is entropy.

Usually, this process requires too much energy to happen, but quantum mechanical "tunneling" acts like a credit line, "lending" molecules enough energy to change forms. Suppose, for example, that a molecule is stable in its normal form and would be stable in a new form, but there is an energy "hill" lying between them. At body temperature, there isn't enough energy to climb the hill. Quantum mechanics says, however, that the temperature actually fluctuates randomly. And very rarely, perhaps once in several decades, the temperature may fluctuate enough to loan energy to a molecule, enabling it to surmount the hill and change into a new molecule. This is extraordinarily rare, but then, the body has such an *enormous* number of molecules that at every moment many of them are spontaneously climbing hills—or, as physicists would say, tunneling through them—somewhere in your body. Your molecules not only rearrange themselves inside your cells, but outside your cells as well—those in the lens of your eye, as you age, for example.

If you wait long enough, any molecule will change. Some will take a day, some months, and some years.[3]

The repair of this spontaneous damage is one of the two reasons you replace (turn over) your molecules continuously; the other is the regulation of the number of molecules (the size of the pool). Of course, this recycling takes energy. It costs you in terms of cellular energy. But that's part of the overhead of being alive. Also, the longer it takes your body to repair the damage, the more likely a wrench will be thrown into the works; the faster you repair the damage, the less likely there will be any long-term effect, but the higher the energy costs will be in continuously active assembly lines.

Damaged molecules can cause even more problems if ignored. The damaged molecule may be needed to make another molecule, which, in turn, would be needed for something else. If damage was done to a gene, the problem is particularly dangerous, because the protein made from that gene also will be damaged, and the process that depended on the protein won't work anymore. Damaged genes are like a company that makes computers that don't work because the plans are faulty. After a while, not only will all the computers be useless, but the company will be out of business. It's no wonder then that your body goes to so much trouble to repair errors in the DNA that makes up your genes.

Isomerization would be bad enough if that was your only problem. Your cells would be saddled with molecules that don't work. Free radicals, however, are worse. Molecules that are damaged by free radicals go on to damage other molecules like a submicroscopic plague. Free radicals are the classic villains in aging. They are a corrosive, they continuously eat away at you, slowly, inexorably taking apart the delicately balanced structures that make up your life.

Free radicals are molecules with a single, unpaired electron in their outermost shell. This electron keeps trying to find a partner, even when it means stealing an electron from, and damaging, other molecules. They do so with haphazard abandon, interfering with normal cell function. Like molecular wolves, they are constantly hungry, latching on to almost any nearby molecule, damaging it by changing its shape and making it useless or dangerous to you. The damaged molecule becomes a misshapen, crippled player on the molecular team. Not only does it no longer function by itself, it interferes with the functioning of its surrounding teammates.

In this way, free radicals are infectious, passing on their unpaired electrons to other victims, which then pass on their electrons, becoming the sources of further damage. The chain of damage extends indefinitely and terminates only when the single electron finds a malevolent mate and settles down, finally and once again at peace. An alternative end to this destructive process occurs when the free radical becomes trapped by a special molecule, a "spin trap" compound, in a relatively stable marriage.

Ironically, the most common free radical in your body is oxygen, an element you cannot do without. Although molecular oxygen is relatively stable, it takes only a very small energy fluctuation[4]—quantum tunneling again—to form single oxygen atoms,[5] which are remarkably reactive with your other molecules.

The location of free radicals contributes to the amount of damage they can cause. Cell membranes, for example, are particularly prone to injury, partly because they are made up of unsaturated fatty acids that are easily oxidized and partly because most free radicals are produced near cell membranes. That increases the amount of damage that radicals can cause, because your membranes are so crucial to cell survival.[6] They are not your only, or even your most important, weak spot, however.

As you age the damage that free radicals do to your DNA library increases.[7] DNA molecules are no more vulnerable than most, but only a limited number of copies of this vital reference library exist, which makes DNA damage more threatening and far more important than

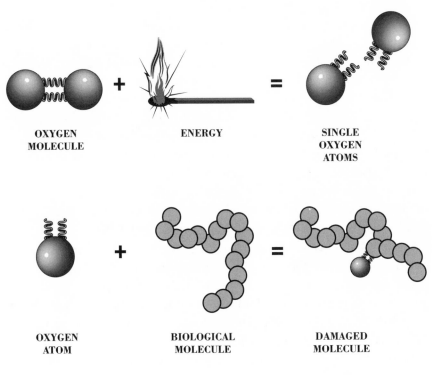

OXYGEN
MOLECULE   +   ENERGY   =   SINGLE
OXYGEN
ATOMS

OXYGEN
ATOM   +   BIOLOGICAL
MOLECULE   =   DAMAGED
MOLECULE

Fig. 2.1

damage to membranes, proteins, or other replaceable components of your cells. Your body can't simply make a new DNA strand from scratch, as it can anything else in your cells. Its only choice is to repair DNA damage.

Why do free radicals exist at all? And why do our cells tolerate these invaders? Because we must have them to survive. Oxygen accounts for 95 percent of our metabolic energy, and we cannot survive without it. Certain forms of oxygen are therefore necessary. We form them continuously in our cells and they are valuable when they are confined safely away from our chromosomes and from other molecules we depend upon. When they escape their bounds, however, as some of them always do, they wreak havoc on nearby molecules. The damage is specific, depending on exactly which free radical gets loose: The solubility, acidity, and proximity to specific sites all determine what gets damaged.

The specific damage is just as dependent on the target: Some amino acids[8] are attacked by free radicals only when hydrogen peroxide interacts with iron, for example. In some cases, damage to DNA, RNA, and proteins may occur only in the presence of normal trace minerals.[9]

The question is not, Can you avoid free radicals? for surely you cannot, but, Can you keep up with the damage? For your germ cells, the answer is yes—they have repaired the damage for several billion years—but what about the rest of your body's cells? How can germ cells do what other cells cannot? Aging cannot simply be a matter of free radicals; perhaps it results from some other type of damage or from damage to specific molecules, such as DNA.

Your DNA library not only holds the entire genetic code for each of your cells, whether germ cell or somatic cell, but encodes all of your repair mechanisms as well. Worse yet, your DNA is subject to a host of specific kinds of entropy that are not faced by your other molecules. Because DNA has the written code for all of your cellular information, because it has the plans for all of your repair procedures, and because it faces special forms of attack by entropy, you devote tremendous effort to the isolating, protecting, and repairing of your DNA. What problems does your DNA face?

It spontaneously falls apart even at body temperature. Not very quickly, but fast enough to be a continuous problem for you. When that happens to other molecules, they can simply be replaced. DNA cannot; it must be repaired flawlessly and quickly moment by moment throughout your life.

The most frequent damage to DNA is to adenine and guanine, two of the four "letters" used in writing your DNA reference books. Parts of these letters split off, leaving only an indecipherable scrawl, as though an eraser randomly eliminated letters from the text in the books that make up your library.

The frequency of this damage is actually quite low: less than one of your letters in 100 quadrillion (1/100,000,000,000,000,000) every day. This is as though a single letter disappeared each day from a single book in a library of a billion volumes. Nonetheless, the human body has so many[10] of these letters in its vast genome library that 5,000 to 10,000 are erased every day. The damage is cumulative and, if not corrected, results in progressive mistakes and, finally, death as normal proteins become replaced by damaged ones. If these changes occur in germ cells, they will accumulate over generations, leading to extinction of any species that allows such damage to persist.

Other DNA damage also occurs. About every fifteen minutes in every one of your trillions of cells, you change As or Cs into other letters entirely—other than the normal four letters, A, C, T, or G; letters not normally used at all in your library. Your genes get misread, the wrong protein is produced and if the cell divides without first erasing the wrong letter and putting the correct letter back in place, the mistake is passed on forever.

These alphabet transplants are caused by your normal body heat, which is simply part of being alive. To quote Pogo: "We have met the enemy and he is us." Your normal body temperature, which you strive diligently to preserve in the face of an often hostile environment, is the culprit. The only way to avoid this continuous damage to your DNA would be to cool yourself to absolute zero. It's true that you would completely cease damaging your DNA, but you wouldn't be alive anymore.

Another source of toxins is your own routine metabolic processes. You intentionally create free radicals, acids, and destructive enzymes and use them to break down and recycle other molecules before they accumulate in dangerous concentrations. These toxins form part of your defenses against viral and bacterial predation, and allow you to generate your metabolic energy. They are metabolic and cellular tools you cannot live without, and yet each one is a source of damage to your DNA, proteins, organelles, and your cells themselves.

The attacks are partly intentional and even necessary for your cells to function. Protein turnover is a normal and reasonable way of assuring that damaged proteins are replaced. You are constantly destroying old proteins and producing new ones. In this case, entropy is in the form of your normal enzymes intentionally tearing down "old" proteins.

DNA receives additional damage from external agents, including high-energy photons and external toxins. High-energy photons—such as cosmic rays, X rays, and ultraviolet light—directly damage the letters in your DNA library or, in the case of cosmic rays, cause harm by ionizing other molecules (which thereby become free radicals) and go on to damage your DNA. The DNA letters form where they shouldn't or split apart in the middle of sentences. Ultraviolet light may cross-link[11] the twin strands of DNA, blocking replication and killing the cell if not repaired. The DNA strand itself can even break, making repair almost impossible.

Cosmic rays are an unavoidable part of life on earth. They constantly bombard our planet and penetrate us. There is nothing we can do to minimize our continual exposure. Ultraviolet light is ubiquitous and only partially avoidable. The major source is the sun. Clothing, sunscreens, buildings (remaining inside), and the melanin in our skin are our only defenses.

Toxins can change the letters in your gene sentences or force themselves between base pairs, adding or subtracting letters and altering genes. They can lock onto both DNA chains, blocking expression when your cell attempts to read the genes. Toxins are often the natural products of other organisms and natural processes; bacteria and plants, for example, produce them as by-products and as defenses against being eaten. Toxins are included in all food, even that unexposed to pesticides and herbicides. It is all but impossible to avoid them: Even a totally synthetic diet contains some toxic molecules and purely "organic" foods certainly do. But food is not the only port of entry. Bacteria and viruses live on your skin and in your intestines, nose, and lungs. These parasites maintain themselves at our expense and are seldom passive players. Antibiotics and our immune systems are only partially effective. The bacteria and viruses stay in our body and burden our immune system; occasionally they even rewrite our genes. These entropic factors are among "the thousand natural shocks that flesh is heir to."

As we ascend from your molecules, cells, tissues, and organs to the level of your entire body, the effects of entropy are present at every level, in occasionally subtle, but always pervasive ways. You are falling apart no matter where you look at yourself. Some of these effects are inherited from a previous, finer level, though some examples are peculiar to certain levels. For instance, your cells inherit damage from the molecular level, but cells also have their own set of entropic demons. Cells inherit and accumulate the results of free radical damage, which involves not only damaged enzymes that must be replaced and damaged DNA that must be repaired, but also waste products. As cells age, many accumulate yellow-brown age pigment (lipofuscin). Certain cells—for example, nerve and heart cells—accumulate quite a bit of this pigment; others—for example, liver cells—don't. In the nervous system, the rate varies by cell type; some cells[12] accumulate lipofuscin when they are young, some more slowly. In general, however, though the rate of accumulation varies remarkably, the correlation with age does not; the older the cell, the more lipofuscin it contains. As you age, you accumulate garbage.

Although the exact composition and sources remain in dispute, lipofuscin derives from oxidized lipids (loosely speaking, partially burned fat molecules). These are, in turn, the products of free radical damage to your membranes. With age, cells have a larger lipofuscin burden to carry. Does this burden harm your cells? No one knows. It is hard to support the notion that these pigments are innocuous, but it is just as difficult to prove that they harm your cells.[13] They probably are a metabolic burden; they almost certainly are an indication of metabolic damage at a finer, molecular level as a result of the mechanisms we have discussed.

Could aging at the cellular level be merely an "inheritance" of the damage that accrues at the molecular level?[14] If so, then not all cells inherit the same amount of damage. Some cells age faster than others, different parts of your body—different tissues—age at different rates. However, your cells continue to function appropriately and efficiently with increasing age by many, but not all, measures. The rate of protein synthesis falls off, for example, while the accuracy of transcription remains high. You produce some proteins more slowly, but just as carefully as ever. Certain genes are repressed, while others are expressed at normal rates. Your cells don't make the same proteins or in the same amounts, but what they *do* produce is normal.

Entropy also occurs not just by inheritance from the molecular level, but *directly* at a higher cellular level. Some of the same agents that were on stage at the biochemical level play a role here as well. Just as normal metabolic heat can cause damage at the molecular level, external heat—or its lack—can cause damage directly at the cellular level. The environment can be either too hot or too cold for cells to survive, or it can be too dry, too salty, too lacking in glucose or other sources of energy, too lacking in oxygen, or too traumatic. Your cells are suited to particular environments and they succumb to insults beyond their design limits. Although a cell rarely suffers noticeably from the enemies that destroy single biological molecules, cells often have their own, larger enemies. For instance, lack of oxygen may not be an immediate problem for a DNA molecule, but it is for a nerve cell; lack of glucose is not a direct problem for RNA, but it is for a heart muscle cell; being hit with a hammer is not fatal to a ribosome, but it is to a skin cell. Each level has its own problems.

Parasites also enter the picture at the cellular level. Viruses that were merely competitive at the molecular level are now fatal enemies. The molecules that translate RNA into proteins may not care whether the RNA is native or viral, but the distinction is a matter of life or death to the cell. Bacteria are irrelevant to the DNA molecule directly, but may kill the heart cell where the DNA lies.

Just as the accumulation of entropic damage at the molecular level affects your cells, cell damage or loss affects your tissues, your organs, your whole body. Cell loss can be catastrophic to the organs or tissues in which it occurs. Loss of a trivial number of cells in the conductance system of your heart may be fatal—and not simply to your heart. Small groups of cells in your brain stem are critical for control of blood pressure, breathing, heart rate, and other vital functions. Your nervous system and many other organs and tissues lose cells, and cell volume, with age.[15] Any loss of cells in one of your critical cell groups affects organ function far beyond the neighborhood of those particular cells. You may sicken or die, becoming the victim of entropic events in small numbers of your cells. Once again, entropic damage at a lower level—cells in this case—can be inherited at higher levels as damage, dysfunction, or even death. At finer levels, the outcome is the alterations to molecules, but at higher levels it is pithy and familiar: disease and death.

Whether the problem is a loss of your cells or an accumulation of molecular abnormalities, most of the aging organs and tissues of your body have similar problems. Cholesterol accumulates in your vessels; plaques are found in Alzheimer's dementia; thinner skin removes the defense against infection; kidneys grow progressively less effective at filtering blood; collagen cross-links and loses elasticity. Attacks occur at all levels and in all organs.

Some of those attacks are traumatic. Skin is worn away by day-to-day abrasion against clothing and the objects we bump into or handle. Lacerations and more energetic abrasions occur when we fall or are hit. Cells and whole areas of skin are torn away and need replacement. Other attacks are infectious. Cells in the lung are killed by a bout of bronchitis or pneumonia, mucosal cells in the nose die from a simple adenovirus as you sniffle and suffer through a cold. HIV attacks and kills white blood cells, leaving its victim defenseless against other infections that, without this loss, would be inconsequential.

At even higher levels, the attacks are to whole systems or entire body (rather than to just cells): the bullet that tears a hole in the aorta, the car that is driven into another oncoming car, the heart going from fifty miles per hour to a complete stop against the inner side of the ribs and rupturing. These represent entropy at a high level.

As I have explained, at any level, you are continuously faced with entropy: Your cells are attacked, and you suffer. Some of those attacks are part of what drives aging, others are incidental or unrelated to it, but all are constant threats to your homeostasis. Any momentary or minimal loss of your defenses increases the threat of dysfunction, disease, and death at some level from your molecules to your entire body.

Under constant threat, you react and defend yourself. You replace, repair, and resist every entropic threat. And, as we will see, you do so with remarkable success.

N E V E R   S U R R E N D E R

We shall fight on the beaches, we shall fight in the fields and in the streets, we shall fight in the hills; we shall never surrender.

—WINSTON CHURCHILL, speech on DUNKIRK

Through the course of evolution—Darwin's natural selection—our genes have been carefully crafted to serve as defenses against the threats we will face in our lifetime. We could say that our defenses have been *designed* to protect us against those threats. But not all organisms need the same defenses. For instance, one organism will have adapted to heat, another to cold; one to life in the water, another to the desert; one to hypoxia, another to too much oxygen. Our genes have adapted to meet the problems we live with. These adaptations are present at the gross level and at the biochemical level.

Entropic dangers differ from organism to organism and, within organism, from cell to cell. For skin cells, ultraviolet exposure—and the free radicals it creates and DNA damage it causes—is of overriding importance and carries a necessarily high metabolic cost to those cells. The priority for the heart muscle cells is the replacement of damaged muscle protein. Skin cells adapt to deal with ultraviolet; heart cells to replace damaged muscle protein. These differences, both among organisms and among cells, determine how aging is expressed. The underlying mechanisms are parallel and often equivalent; the outcome is varied and correlates with these, and innumerable other, differences among cells and among organisms.

We vigorously defend ourselves against whatever attack we face. At every level, we have specific ways of doing so by minimizing, avoiding, replacing, or repairing damage. For example, when proteins are damaged, your body increases the turnover, thereby diluting the ineffective ones. This process is, of course, expensive in terms of hard-earned metabolic energy, which you cannot afford to waste. There is a constant turnover of molecules—proteins and others as well—which increases if the damage rate goes up. In special cases—DNA, for instance—turnover is not feasible, and repair is the only option.

Most proteins can be replaced because the DNA template is available to create new copies ad infinitum. DNA, however, is its own template and, as stated earlier, can only be repaired. In fact, DNA is the only large biological molecule capable of being repaired after it has sustained structural damage.[16] But it can only be repaired if the repair machinery knows what the original molecule was. If a base letter is missing on one strand, but the letter opposite it is a thymine, we know that the missing letter must be adenine because adenine always pairs with thymine. To repair the DNA, your body would weld an adenine into the hole in the DNA chain. Then your chromosome and your cell would be able to go on.

The body also has paired chromosomes, made of DNA, but although the genes on each chromosome generally correspond, they are rarely an exact match because each of them came from a different parent. The pairing of chromosomes does provide some measure of safety. If the hemoglobin gene you inherit from one parent is damaged, but the gene you receive from the other parent is normal, in most cases the faulty gene will be merely ineffective. If both parents provide a sickle-cell gene, the abnormal hemoglobin will form clumps that distort your red blood cells into sickle-shaped cells that become lodged in your smaller capillaries. Those clumps of cells block blood flow and kill your tissues, as happens on sickle-cell anemia.

DNA repair is continuous and all but flawless. The process is complex, requiring multiple steps and instructions from multiple genes, each of which is itself subject to repair. In every case, the repair must occur rapidly so that the process does not suffer from genetic damage. It takes little imagination to picture the vicious cycle that might ensue if DNA were not repaired quickly. For instance, if one of your DNA repair genes is faulty, then damaged DNA could be transcribed into flawed RNA, which would then be translated into a flawed enzyme. That enzyme would then try to repair the damaged DNA, but it would botch the job, creating additional errors rather than correcting the original ones. The cycle would occur again, with even more errors in the DNA. And with each cycle the damage would spread until a substantial portion of the chromosome became involved or until some vital protein, produced from the damaged DNA, failed and the cell finally died.

Generally, there are two types of DNA repair that occur. In the first, and least common kind, the damaged letter is left in place and repaired where it is. That is the norm when an abnormal molecule has been added to the DNA, and also in cases when dimer formation has occurred. (DNA dimers—in which DNA bases stick to one another when they should be separated—are a normal and continuous form of damage that results from even low-level exposure to sunlight. A mutation of any one of the genes that are responsible for fixing DNA dimers[17] will prevent normal repair and cause xeroderma pigmentosa, a disease that makes one prone to cancers, chronic pain, and early death. The body has at least nine separate repair genes devoted to this damage.)

The more common method of repair is by excision and replacement. DNA repair enzymes, a separate one for each step, are responsible for fixing the damaged DNA. The abnormal letters must be cut free of their neighbors and then removed and a new letter synthesized and then reattached. Not only is the process complex, but each DNA letter has a different set of repair enzymes; if any of those enzymes doesn't work, then the attempt to repair damaged DNA will either be ineffective or cause even more damage. At any stage in the process, there are enormous opportunities for mutational error and loss of normal gene expression, with clinical consequences, such as age-related diseases.

A potential problem in this process can be overly efficient DNA repair. For instance, if the repair enzymes are not well regulated or are too nonspecific in their targets, they may repair "mistakes" that were not errors at all. They may blithely excise regions of intentional modifications that the cell has made to control gene expression[18] or has used to generate novel antibodies. This happens quite rarely, however.

Not only do you repair your DNA and turn over molecules such as proteins and lipids you don't repair, but your body also takes steps to avoid damage in the first place.[19] Damage from free radicals, for example, is prominent during aging. The body's mechanisms that defend against free radicals are at least as complex as those that deal with repairing damage. They employ four different strategies: They lock up the free radicals, make proteins to trap and metabolize them, rely on other (nonprotein) molecules to trap them,[20] and replace the molecules that they damage. Locking up the free radicals occurs by isolating them in cellular compartments away from other parts of the cell, particularly away from DNA. Trapping is accomplished by proteins that the cell produces, such as superoxide dismutase (SOD), which then metabolize the free radicals to something less dangerous. Not all trapping of free radicals is done by proteins that the cell makes: Trapping can also be accomplished by molecules that the cell imports from your diet (vitamin E, for example). The fourth method of defense is simply to turn over damaged molecules and replace them with new ones. Let's look at each method in turn.

Most free radicals are produced and kept locked up in the mitochondria, the power stations responsible for transforming energy into usable forms for your cells. The mitochondria break down glucose and form a molecule—ATP (adenosine triphosphate)—which is the standard currency for most of the cellular economy. Any time your cells do anything that costs energy, the bill is likely to be aid in ATP, and your mitochondria will have printed the currency. Besides making energy, your mitochondria are like power stations in another way as well: Like nuclear power plants, they are isolated from the cellular neighborhood by a set of membrane walls. The result is relative protection of your

DNA. For every several hundred thousand free radicals, only one damages your DNA.[21]

Although most free radicals are found in your mitochondria,[22] they are also present in small amounts throughout the cell, and they occur spontaneously. Because of this, the cell has two other forms of protection short of giving up and replacing the damage. The body produces proteins that are specifically designed to trap free radicals, and it has other, nonprotein molecules, usually dietary molecules (such as vitamin E and other tocopherols), that also trap free radicals.

Most important in trapping free radicals—from the perspective of aging and its reversal—are your protective enzymes, including superoxide dismutase (SOD), catalase, and glutathione peroxidase. Together those three enzymes not only trap but metabolize free radicals: Starting with an unpaired oxygen atom, for example, these enzymes can produce innocuous and useful molecules, such as water, as an end product. The best-known of these enzymes, SOD, is actually a family of enzymes. These SODs first turn certain oxygen radicals and hydrogen into hydrogen peroxide and oxygen, terminating the free radical chain of reactions. Catalase, (CAT), probably the second most important free-radical-trapping protein after SOD, acts in tandem with the SOD family of enzymes, turning the hydrogen peroxide into oxygen and water. A third free-radical-trapping protein, glutathione peroxidase, acts in a somewhat similar fashion, also reducing hydrogen peroxide to water. The reaction starts with free radicals and ends with normal, paired oxygen molecules—not free radicals anymore—and water. The unpaired electrons—free radicals—combine into molecules that are no longer dangerous. Your cells regulate how much of each of these enzymes is present, and that governs to a large extent, how much damage occurs.

The effectiveness of each enzyme also dictates how much damage occurs. There is a linear correlation between the efficiency of these enzymes and the typical life span of a species. Human beings, having long life spans, produce extraordinarily effective SOD in sufficient concentrations to cope with all but a tiny fraction of their free radicals. The enzymes work quite well, but no matter how many or how efficient they are, a certain number of free radicals will still exist long enough, or in high enough concentrations, to damage your other molecules.

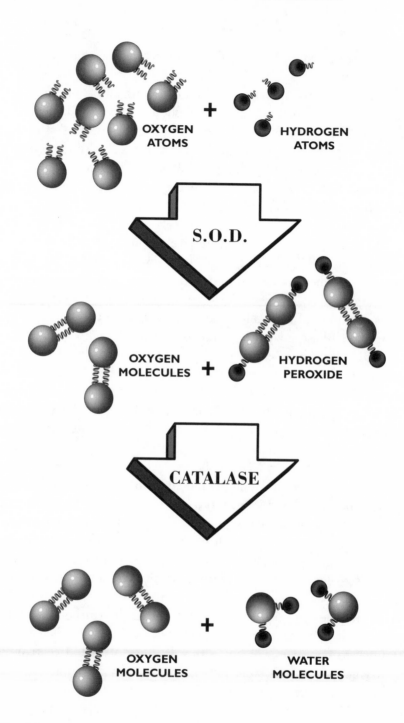

OXYGEN ATOMS + HYDROGEN ATOMS

S.O.D.

OXYGEN MOLECULES + HYDROGEN PEROXIDE

CATALASE

OXYGEN MOLECULES + WATER MOLECULES

Fig. 2.2

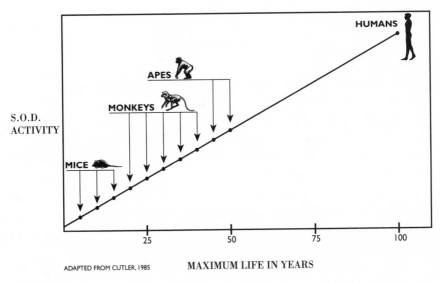

ADAPTED FROM CUTLER, 1985   **MAXIMUM LIFE IN YEARS**

Fig. 2.3

Also playing a prominent role in the defense against free radicals are nonenzymatic compounds. The majority of these (for example, as vitamins E and C), but not all (urate and melatonin are exceptions)[23] come from your diet. They act as sinks for free radicals. After they absorb the extra electron from the free radical thereby preventing a chain reaction of damage, they can either be regenerated or excreted and replaced. The nonenzymatic compounds are a large family of molecules, including glutathione, ascorbic acid (vitamin C), urate, melatonin, tocopherols (vitamin E, especially alphatocopherol), ubiquinones, and carotenoids.[24] Most of these are present in your diet. Antioxidant molecules such as vitamin E, ascorbate, and the carotenoids have become the supplement of choice for many people wishing to lessen their risk of coronary artery disease and death.

These antioxidant molecules are expendable and replaceable as they wage war on free radicals. You can simply ingest more of them. They are largely regulated by intestinal absorption, by the abundance of free radicals in the cell and, in some cases, by how many such antioxidant molecules your cells produce. Their concentrations may be low because of poor availability—for instance, when the diet is poor or absorption is limited—or because of an abundance of free radicals—the more antioxidants are used in eliminating free radicals, the fewer will remain.

The clearest evidence that these nonenzymatic compounds protect you from damage by free radicals can be seen in lipofuscin, the aging pigment found in cells that probably consists of partially oxidized fat molecules. The amount of lipofuscin accumulation depends on the species, the tissue, the age, and to some extent the diet. Specifically, it depends on the dietary intake of certain scavengers that consume free radicals, such as vitamin E. For instance, when the diet is deficient in vitamin E, there will be greater accumulations of lipofuscin.

What happens when we add antioxidants in an attempt to extend the life span? Though we can increase the average life span we have not usually been able to lengthen the maximum life span, although even that has been done in some species.[25] We can increase the average animal's chances of surviving into old age, but we can't alter old age itself. Although dietary supplementation does result in decreased accumulation of oxidized lipids in general and lipofuscin in particular, this generally still does not retard aging.[26] Free radical scavengers alone won't stop you from aging.

The cell might even need small amounts of free radicals to work normally and might intentionally maintain their level. So adding antioxidant compounds in supernormal amounts can do more than just affect the lipofuscin concentrations.[27] Free radical damage, while crucial to understanding aging at the metabolic level, is a secondary phenomenon; it is regulated, monitored, and even necessary, but not itself the primary control for aging.[28]

If all of these traps are ineffective (and to some degree they are, and—as the last paragraph suggests—should be), your cells have the final option of living with the continuous damage and simply destroying the damaged molecule and replacing it with a newly synthesized one. But replacement still leaves you with two problems: (1) It is expensive—it takes energy to continuously rebuild molecules. In the ultimate case, if you used all your cellular energy (ATP from your mitochondria) to rapidly make and as rapidly destroy molecules all day, there would be no ATP left to enable you to move, eat, or defend yourself against infection. Since your body needs ATP to do all of those things, and everything else, you can't afford to replace your molecules too quickly. (2) Some of the damaged molecules—such as lipofuscin—accumulate in the cells rather than being recycled.

Free radicals are certainly not your only enemy. Not only does your body repair damage from free radicals; it also repairs changes caused by isomerization. The enzymes responsible for this repair, like those that defend against free radicals, are found in each of your cells, and their availability—but not their activity—declines with age, especially after you reach the age of forty.[29] It is less clear how, if at all, your body repairs damage to proteins outside the cell. There is reason to think that it does, however—though it becomes less and less efficient at it as time goes by.

We have looked at entropic forces that actively attempt to destroy your molecules, your cells, and your entire body, and have examined the defenses the body uses to ward off the destruction. But how do these two opposing forces strike a balance, and how do they finally lose that balance and tip you toward aging?

THE BALANCE AND THE WAR

Turning and turning in a widening gyre
The falcon cannot hear the falconer;
Things fall apart; the center cannot hold;
Mere anarchy is loosed upon the world.

—WILLIAM BUTLER YEATS, "THE SECOND COMING"

Life is a constant war. At every moment we are engaged in a struggle against isomers, free radicals, infections, starvation, other species, or too often, each other. When we lose any of these battles at any level—biochemical, cellular, systemic, or in the whole organism—death occurs. At every level, life is balanced between entropy and defense, degradation and restoration; when this balance is lost, aging occurs. Therefore, the only way to reverse aging is to restore the balance.

But in some cases, the key to reversing aging is not so much the balance as the rate of turnover. For instance, your body builds new protein molecules as quickly as it loses them. As you age, your ability to synthesize proteins is as faithful and accurate as it always was, but there are more damaged proteins because they simply aren't recycled as fast as they were when you were young. As a result, the damaged proteins linger. The size of the pool of each protein molecule is determined by the balance between their degradation and the synthesis of new, undamaged protein.

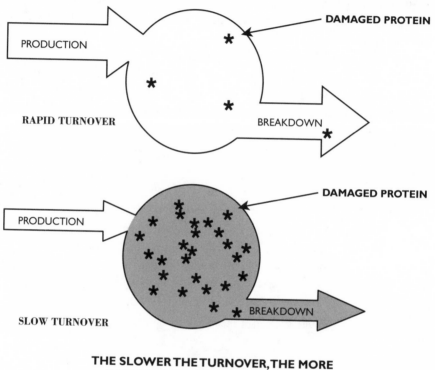

THE SLOWER THE TURNOVER, THE MORE DAMAGED PROTEINS ACCUMULATE

Fig. 2.4

The process of breakdown and production can be fast or slow, but as long as they are equal in measure, the pool size will stay the same. If the turnover is high, but both degradation and renewal remain equal, damaged proteins will be rapidly replaced by new, normal ones. If the turnover is low, with both breakdown and production equally slow, the pool size will remain the same, but proteins will remain in the pool longer, and it is more likely that they will be damaged by free radicals, isomerization, or a host of other enemies. Once damaged, the protein sits in the pool until your cell finally gets around to breaking it down.

It might be assumed that the cell breaks down only damaged proteins, but it can't tell them apart well enough, so it recycles all of them, and the faster it does it, the fewer damaged ones there will be.

Pools—collections of items, such as particular molecules or types of cells—are common in biology and are a useful concept in understanding aging. There are pools of proteins, pools of lipids, even pools of cells. The size of the pool tells us how many molecules are available; the turnover rate and the damage rate together indicate how many of those molecules are still functional.

For some of the proteins in our cells, the pool size decreases with aging. That is particularly true of important regulatory proteins, such as those controlling how fast other proteins are produced. In most cases, however, the pool size doesn't seem to change much with aging, although the turnover rates slow and the concentration of damaged molecules increases. Your pool of red blood cells is replenished constantly. Their average life span is 120 days; almost 1 percent of your red cells are replaced each day.[30] When you lose blood, you accelerate production until the pool size returns to normal; if you are given extra blood, production slows until the pool size is again normal.

The red blood cell membranes constitute yet another pool, made up of lipid molecules that "age." Red blood cells do not manufacture proteins nor do they replace damaged membranes. Entropy is allowed to have its way, and the cell fades to a passive death. If your body does not remove "old" red cells from your blood—a properly functioning spleen usually does that for you—the concentration of damaged red cells rises even though the pool size stays constant.[31]

The cells of your skin, intestinal lining, blood vessel walls, immune system, all have pools that are constantly being replenished. Turnover is necessary for most of your molecules, but the slower the turnover, the less effective any pool will be. The pool size of some molecules may decrease as you age, but even if the pool is constant, it will have a higher concentration of damaged molecules if the turnover is slower.

Turnover becomes slower as we age; protein synthesis declines by more than one half;[32] so does the rate of protein breakdown, so the pool sizes remain fairly constant. Our cells just don't recycle as well as they once did. The result is an increased number of damaged proteins in the pool even without any production errors or any increase in the rate of damage.

Imagine a garden with one hundred plants in it, and that once a day the owner randomly pulls up fifty of the plants and puts in fifty healthy, new ones. Every night you—as an agent of entropy—sneak in and destroy just one of the plants. Every day there is a 50-percent chance the damaged plant will be taken out as one of the fifty plants that the owner removes and a 100-percent chance that it will be replaced by a healthy plant (since that's all the owner ever puts in the garden). Over time, as we settle into our roles, there will be an average of two damaged plants on any particular day. Some days there may be a few more, some days there may be none, but on the average there will be two dead plants.

Now what would happen should the garden's owner become lazy? Assume that every day he now puts in only two new plants instead of fifty, and takes out only two. Assume that you continue to damage only one each night. Now, over time, the number of damaged plants will increase to an average of half (50/100) of all the plants.[33] The damage rate hasn't changed, but the turnover has slowed and the number of damaged plants increased. As it does with molecules.

This is part of what happens as we age. The rate of adding plants (protein production) and subtracting plants (protein degradation) fall simultaneously. The number of plants in the garden (the protein pool) and the rate at which they are damaged (the rate of protein damage) can remain constant, but the result will still be an increase in the number of dead plants (the number of damaged proteins in your protein pool). As we grow older, the percentage of damaged molecules rises, because the turnover slows, even if the damage rate doesn't change at all.

The role of decreasing turnover is important in aging, but it is still far from being the entire story. DNA is not renewed in the same way as are proteins; instead, it is unique in being repaired rather than replaced. Similar problems still occur, however. DNA repair must be both effective and rapid. If repair is only partial, even if done quickly, it will result in more and more partially repaired DNA errors that in turn result in faulty proteins and, ultimately, the death of your cells. Slower repair, even if complete, increases the chances that your cells will read from as yet unrepaired DNA—and produce damaged protein as a result—before your enzymes get around to fixing the DNA damage. If the flawed protein made from the still-unrepaired DNA is itself normally supposed to be part of the DNA repair process, then the

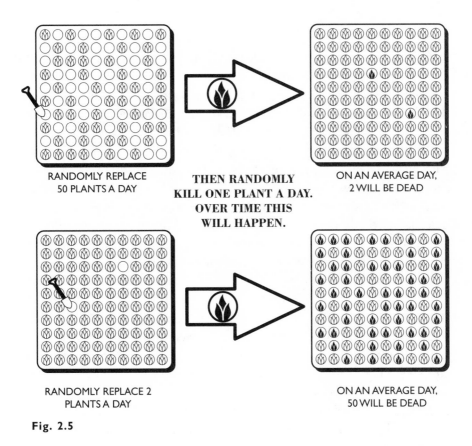

RANDOMLY REPLACE
50 PLANTS A DAY

**THEN RANDOMLY
KILL ONE PLANT A DAY.
OVER TIME THIS
WILL HAPPEN.**

ON AN AVERAGE DAY,
2 WILL BE DEAD

RANDOMLY REPLACE 2
PLANTS A DAY

ON AN AVERAGE DAY,
50 WILL BE DEAD

Fig. 2.5

process will feed on itself: The still-unrepaired DNA will manufacture damaged repair proteins, which won't repair DNA correctly, the percentage of flawed DNA will increase, and the percentage of damaged proteins will increase. As time passes, your cells will have more and more difficulty making repairs as they read from damaged DNA. The center of the cell, the DNA, will gradually accumulate errors, "turning and turning in a widening gyre . . . ," until the growing number of errors are lethal to your cells and finally to you.

A slower turnover rate, in the case of proteins, lipids, etc., or a slower or inadequate repair, in the case of DNA, will become a progressive problem for the cell, separating cells into "the quick and the dead."

The process of turnover and DNA repair deal with the problems of molecular damage. An equally important factor, however, is the rate at which damage occurs. At first thought, that appears to be constant:

How can the concentration of free radicals vary? It can vary in two ways, through production and degradation. Just as molecules exist in a pool, so too do free radicals, and they too are influenced by production and degradation (in the case of free radicals, trapping by antioxidants). The larger the pool of free radicals, the more damage they can cause in each of your cells; the smaller the pool, the less the damage.

Production varies from time to time—but probably not very much with age—depending on your exposure to toxins and high-energy photons as well as on your normal metabolism. On the other hand, trapping of free radicals never quite keeps up with production[34] and your defenses certainly decrease with age.[35] In addition, free radicals are not confined within your mitochondria as well when you age; the mitochondrial barriers, made of lipid membranes, weaken with age, and you begin to leak.

Let's look more carefully at each of the three ways—production, trapping, and confinement—in which the availability of free radicals might change as aging occurs. The first factor is free radical production. Although there has been some dispute in this regard,[36] Byung Yu, an expert in the field at the University of Texas, has stated that free radical *production* does not increase as you age.[37] That is not to say, however, that free radical *concentration* or pool size does not increase with age. In fact, it does exactly that, apparently owing to the decrease in availability or efficacy—or both—of antioxidants as you age.[38] Free-radical-trapping compounds are less abundant and less effective. Essentially, you produce the same number of free radicals but you trap fewer of them; as a result, the pool of available free radicals increases with age, and that increase leads to more frequent damage to your cells.

The third factor (confinement within your mitochondria) probably changes as well. Not only does your body have more free radicals to deal with as you age, but it becomes less effective at confining them. Mitochondria[39] are the classic examples of membrane-bound, localized producers of free radicals.[40] As we age, free radicals damage lipid membranes, making them more permeable.[41] If free radicals do enough damage to their boundaries, they are able to escape and attack the rest of our cells.

Although the damaged membranes are replaced, the recycling is never total. Some "garbage"—lipofuscin, for example—accumulates over time and may interfere with cell function. Worse yet, our ability to rid the body of damaged lipids declines as we age.[42] We are caught in a tightening noose.

The very mechanisms that are needed to defend against free radicals are themselves sustaining damage. For example, the increase in free radicals accelerates the deterioration of the lipid membranes that confine the free radicals, of proteins (some of which are free radical traps), and of nucleic acids (including the very genes that code for your defenses). This damage increases exponentially with aging, as our defenses become the targets of free radicals. Entropy, or, as Yeats said, "mere anarchy" is loosed upon our cells.

It is not surprising, then, that species with long life spans have high levels of defenses against free radicals—and vice versa.[43] Those defenses are what primarily stand between an organism and entropic dissolution. An organism's life is a moment-to-moment battle between homeostasis and entropy. However, although some have argued that entropic forces themselves—for example, free radicals—are responsible for every aspect of aging, including its triggering, there is more to aging than simply entropic damage per se, and perhaps a great deal more, as we may learn when we explore the underlying mechanisms that allow this damage to occur.

As is evident, the damage begins and proceeds to its conclusion at different times and at different rates in various organisms. If our germ cells have the same genes as our somatic cells—though expressed differently—and share the same environment, why don't they age in the same way? After all, they have the same aging membranes, the same problem with metabolic waste accumulation, the same free radical damage. In what way are germ cells so special that they avoid aging while apparently identical somatic cells age and die? That question arises repeatedly and we must answer it before we can understand how aging actually begins. All the entropic forces (free radicals, isomerization, decreased turnover, etc.) alone are not enough to cause aging. There is also some switch that lets loose those forces within most of your cells, but not within your germ cells. Thus, there must be more to aging than Yeats's "mere anarchy"; there must be something that *lets loose* anarchy upon your cells.

To truly understand what causes aging, the absolutely critical questions are what triggers the decline, and why does it begin when it does? Even if we understand the decline itself to some degree, why does it begin when it does? Why does each species have a different life span? These lead to the ultimate question, why don't we live forever? Or, better phrased, why do we age and die?[44] Why should we? Above all, and most important, to you, what can we do to reverse the process?

It is not surprising that we don't live forever.

Aging, on the other hand, is a different matter. As already noted, a host of entropic factors provide the driving force toward a final dissolution, but some cells hold them at bay indefinitely. Germ cells, and many one-celled organisms, fend them off constantly and permanently. Therefore, aging requires a trigger, some factor that looses the dogs of time, allowing entropy free rein to destroy and undermine the body. Free radicals are crucial in this process: They are the hounds that take you down, but what sets them loose?

The facts that some species—and all germ lines—are immortal and that mortal species age and die at different rates, strongly suggest that aging originates in the genes. Your genes define your life span both through the efficiency of your defenses against free radicals and through the leash that holds these agents at bay. Where in your genes is your life span set? The clock that defines your *maximum* life span is located in at most only a few genes.[45]

The *actual* life span of an organism is, of course, determined by many factors. The actual living out of that span is quite astoundingly complex: Literally every gene plays some role in it. All of your genes are involved in maintaining homeostasis and resisting entropy, but only a few genes determine when you actually stop *trying* to maintain such homeostasis and let entropy have its way.

Whatever it is, and wherever it lies within you, this master switch affects the key points in your cells. It represses the genes that control your defenses against free radicals; the genes controlling crucial parts of your cellular metabolism, including protein production (and the turnover rate within protein pools); and the genes responsible for DNA repair—although the majority of genes are unaffected by the aging process.

When that switch is thrown, the result is a widespread increase in damage as you age, the overall outcome being a loss of balance. No longer are your homeostatic mechanisms balanced against the continual entropic damage, but your homeostatic defenses are gradually turned off and you slowly lose the battles in every important arena of the metabolic war.

Skirmishes continue in the countryside, but the decisive battle has been lost; your troops have left the field, the day fades, and the night slowly descends. The war is over. Aging progresses, and death is the final outcome. Initially, the loss of balance is minimal and barely detectable, but soon the outcome is overwhelming and obvious. The genes themselves slowly and deliberately open the gates and invite entropy in. Aging is subtle, but pervasive; it "creeps in this petty pace from day to day, to the last syllable of recorded time."[46] To understand such a process, let's consider two sorts of aging that are not subtle at all: aging within cells and aging in children with progeria.

OLD CELLS, OLD CHILDREN

"Death," said I, "what do you here
At this Spring season of the year?"
"I mark the flowers ere the prime
Which I may tell at Autumn-time."

—GERARD MANLEY HOPKINS,
"SPRING AND DEATH"

It was not until well past the middle of this century that we came to realize that cells themselves have definite and characteristic life spans.[47] Not only do organisms have a life span specific to each species, but within each organism, cells have their own life spans: a limit on how many times that type of cell may divide. Could the limit for a cell be part of what determines the life span of the organism made up of such cells? Perhaps we might find our clock for aging by looking into cells that age. Perhaps both cells and organisms have the same trigger.

As we learned in Chapter 1, prior to Leonard Hayflick's work many scientists had believed that any cell could be kept alive to divide in-definitely with careful tissue culture, but they were wrong. The first—

and classic—experiment in which cell senescence was demonstrated was conducted on fibroblasts. This common type of cell can be taken from your upper arm with a small punch biopsy (which removes a quarter-inch plug of skin), separated from other cells, and allowed to grow in a culture dish in the laboratory. Although cells can divide and survive for varying amounts of time depending on their type and culture conditions, cells that are allowed to divide will invariably undergo a finite and reproducible number of divisions before senescing and finally dying. This "Hayflick limit" is specific—and different—for each type of cell and for each species. The limit on the number of generations of cells is invariable and has been unaffected by any laboratory interventions until now. There is something that counts the generations and reliably triggers cell senescence. There is a clock.

If, as Hayflick did, we grow fibroblasts in culture until the cells have doubled, then divide them in half and do it again, each "doubling" is a generation of cells. When the cells will no longer divide (and show other indications of cell senescence), they have reached their Hayflick limit. The maximum number of generations can be obtained from fetal donors, for example, from placental tissue. Cultures taken of fibroblasts from older donors result in fewer generations for the same types of cells. As you age, your fibroblasts have already undergone some of their limited number of divisions and are that much closer to their Hayflick limits. The clock that determines the limit has run down.

In a general way, the Hayflick limit of a cell is determined by three things: the maximum life span of the species from which it was drawn; the proportion of that life span that the donor has already lived (the age of the donor); and the cell type, each cell type (fibroblasts, white blood cells, etc.) having its own Hayflick limit. Both the life span in a species and aging in your own body are correlated with the Hayflick limit of the cells. Perhaps the triggers for aging in both the cells and the entire body are the same as well.

What happens if the trigger is released too early? What if the clock, whatever it is, runs down too fast? That is what occurs in progeria ("early aging") syndromes, which are as tantalizing and provocative to consider as the Hayflick limit. In these syndromes, aging seems to occur far earlier than for most of us, as though the switch has been thrown too early. The two most interesting (because we know more about them and they shed the most light on aging) are the Hutchinson-

Gilford syndrome (sometimes simply called progeria) and Werner's syndrome.

Hutchinson-Gilford syndrome was first described in 1886. Children with Hutchinson-Gilford syndrome are extraordinarily rare (one in eight million births[48]) but haunting and unforgettable. The child typically shows symptoms during the first year of life and generally dies by age thirteen of what looks for all the world to be overwhelming old age. Werner's syndrome is only slightly more common (probably one in several million births[49]). It typically appears during the twenties and most who suffer from it die, apparently because of old age, by age fifty.

Both of these diseases manifest themselves as what appears to be accelerated aging. The patients may show early cataracts, "old" skin, facial changes typical of the elderly, gray hair or balding, heart disease, strokes, and aneurysms. That aging itself is difficult to pin down has made it easy to argue that neither of these "progeric" syndromes is anything of the kind, but rather represents a different disease process altogether that merely mimics some of the superficial characteristics of normal aging. This is not a bootless argument. There are some clear differences between progeric aging and normal aging. For example, although Hutchinson-Gilford patients typically demonstrate early cardiovascular disease and a high frequency of death from myocardial infarction—common for aged patients—they do not demonstrate correspondingly increased cholesterol accumulation, lipofuscin accumulation, or hypertension. Likewise, their rates and types of cancer do not correspond with their apparently advanced age. Osteoporosis and other bony changes, such as arthritis, that typically occur with normal aging have a different distribution in these children.[50]

Despite this, clinical observation and the majority of published opinions on the question suggest that these two diseases are closely related to aging and pertinent to an understanding of the underlying process. Very few would argue that the two syndromes are totally unrelated to aging. The crux of the argument is at what stage of the aging mechanism these diseases act and whether they can provide insight into that mechanism.

To the extent that progeria is an accelerated form of aging, the implications are that aging is not simply a process of wear and tear or of entropy. Rather, just as in the case of aging cells in culture, there is a clock, but one that is awry and permits entropy to run its course prematurely. Progeria teaches us that aging is not a passive process, but one that is triggered and at a far younger age in progeric children than in most of us.

But how can we be sure that it is early aging at all? Does progeria simply employ a few of the final common pathways of normal aging, causing a cosmetic resemblance—or is the error actually at the deepest level—resetting the underaging clock—and does the outcome vary from normal aging only because it acts on a different substrate?

Certainly, in the case of Hutchinson-Gilford syndrome, the six-month-old provides a quite different origin on which the aging process can act than does the normal substrate of the mature human; we would be extraordinarily naive to expect an identical outcome even if the "vector" that acts on it were identical. If the process of aging begins earlier—and even if it employs an identical mechanism—the final outcome will be different because the mechanism began its work at a different age and on a markedly different organism than is normally the case. This will be especially true of the Hutchinson-Gilford children. Aging in these children can be expected to differ radically from normal aging given the marked lack of development in the organism on which aging works its destruction. Given the difference in substrate (child versus adult), it is remarkable that Hutchinson-Gilford syndrome resembles normal aging to any degree at all, yet the parallels remain striking. To a lesser degree, the same argument can be made with Werner's syndrome, causing age to manifest decades earlier than is normal, although on an adult organism rather than a young child.

With these caveats, let us consider some of the implications of Hayflick limits and progerias for understanding the mechanisms of aging. Since cells can only divide a limited number of times, the logical conclusion would seem to be that we age because we simply run out of cells. However, that is not the case at all. To begin with, we generally don't run out of cells. For example, we can culture fibroblasts from humans of any age, even centenarians, and, although the cells have fewer generations before dying, they still grow and divide. We can find viable fibroblasts in people of any age. There is no age so advanced that it precludes cells being cultured and made to divide. The clock does not simply arrive at midnight and stop. Older cells are slow to divide and they are abnormal in many ways, but at least a few of our cells can still divide at any age.

But why should we expect it to be otherwise? The reason that the person is still alive for us to sample may be that their fibroblasts, and many other cells, are still capable of dividing and living. If all their cells were incapable of dividing anymore, wouldn't the person be dead in the first place? The fact that the older person has not "run out of cells" is not surprising then.

On the other hand, many older people have almost run out of cells; there may be insufficient cells to function well and to defend them against entropy. No longer can they fend off infection and trauma. In the skin alone, the defensive barriers have thinned, and regrowth after injury is slow and limited in extent, just as their growth of fibroblasts is slow and limited. But how does this affect the body as a whole?

Consider a house, held together by nails. If each day we remove a few nails one by one, carefully pulling them out so that every day there are fewer, what happens? The house will do well for a while, seemingly strong and sound. Then, one day, a gust of wind will free up a board here or there, a few shingles will fly away, the rain will find its way through, a wall will sag. The days pass, and we continue to pull a nail here and another there. With little warning, one day the house collapses and "dies." Does the house still have nails? Yes, but not enough. Does the centenarian still have cells capable of dividing? Yes, but not enough.

The "trigger" of the collapsing house is our pulling nails. The "trigger" in aging is something within each cell, something that determines the Hayflick limit, and that determines when a cell is old. It is something subtle, which "pulls the nails" from our cells. It is ironic perhaps that the house collapses, still with some nails left, tight and strong; it is ironic as well that the body dies, still with some normal cells, capable and efficient. But not quite capable and efficient enough for the final stress that brought it down.

Is it just a matter of nails, then? Is aging just a loss of cells? No, it is more complex, and yet, the loss of the ability of cells to replicate and perform their normal functions is crucial to clinical aging. Without those cells, the body can no longer defend and renew itself in the face of entropy. The cell's loss of ability to divide and the cell's decreasing function is pivotal in understanding the diseases of aging. This is true of the fibroblasts in your skin, the endothelial cells that line your blood vessels, and the white blood cells that fight infections. The aneurysm ruptures, the heart muscle loses its blood supply and dies, and the immune system is overwhelmed by otherwise trivial infections. Unexpectedly, the organism succumbs and often dies, as though without cause. Yet there is cause: a subtle loss of sufficient cells and, more important, an inability of those that remain to perform crucial functions. Although the loss is gradual and cumulative, the outcome is sudden, without warning, and too often fatal.

But why do these cells have fewer divisions left? What is the mechanism that counts those divisions and allots so few to older cells? The answers will prove to have profound consequences not only for our understanding of aging, but for our ability to alter or even reverse it. If we are to answer these questions, we must know what we mean by aging.

LOSING THE TRUST

O chestnut-tree, great-rooted blossomer,
Are you the leaf, the blossom or the bole?
O body swayed to music, O brightening glance,
How can we know the dancer from the dance?

—WILLIAM BUTLER YEATS, "AMONG SCHOOL CHILDREN"

Aging is an intrinsic, cumulative, and inevitable loss of function causing a progressive increase in the potential for disease and death. Ultimately, your chances of survival become zero in the face of declining biological function and increasing susceptibility to disease. None of us has ever been immune to aging, none has ever survived the process.

At a deeper level, the question of the *mechanism* of aging remains; or, in merely descriptive terms, the *cause* of aging still eludes us. The cause has been difficult to discern among a wealth of clinical and biochemical data. We see small pieces of the whole, but fail to understand how they make up the whole process of aging. We look so closely at "the leaf, the blossom, or the bole," that we miss the tree itself. What is aging? Is it merely the increase in damage by free radicals, the weakening in immune function, the increased likelihood of DNA damage, or slower protein turnover? While it is all of these things, and many more, it is also something else.

There is something greater, more subtle, or deeper than any of these causes of aging. Clinically and scientifically, we have, over the years, come to know the "dancers," but we have yet to understand the "dance." Comprehending the underlying cause of aging will likely allow us to alter the process. But we must separate the underlying cause of aging from the effects. It would be insufficient to remove cholesterol plaques, lower blood pressure, make collagen more elastic, prevent cross-linking, reverse isomerization, scavenge free radicals, and increase protein turnover. If we could deal with *all these secondary phenomena simultaneously*, we could prevent the *expression* of aging; we would not have dealt with the actual cause.

Even if we removed all free radical damage, you would still age because there are other entropic mechanisms responsible for cumulative damage within your cells. If we took away isomerization and high-energy photons and removed all DNA damage, you would still age. These factors, and dozens of others, are interactive, cumulative, and sufficient for aging, but eliminating any one of them would not prevent aging. These are mechanisms that drive aging, but not the cause, the trigger, the primary mechanism, the timer; they are not the clock.

THE GARDEN

Our bodies are our gardens, to the which our wills are gardeners.

—*OTHELLO*, I.iii

Again, let's consider the example of a garden. If you spend time planting, weeding, pruning, mulching, fertilizing, and watering your plants, your garden will be healthy. You can ignore the garden for several years, and then blame the result on weeds, lack of water, insects, animals, or disease, but it will fall apart because it lacked a caretaker. If you don't take care of the garden, entropy triumphs. The degeneration of your garden is not caused by the weeds, but by the lack of weeding. The mechanism that started the process was the firing of the gardener; the problem was the neglect of weeding, rather than the weeds that result.

Aging is initiated by changes in gene expression as we grow older. We repress the genes that control free radicals,—which were present long before we began aging—rather than changing the free radicals themselves. The question is who is the caretaker and why was he fired? A more pressing question is, perhaps, can we hire another equally qualified caretaker.

The "caretaker" is an appropriate metaphor here. All of your homeostatic mechanisms are, in a sense, individual gardeners, carefully tending portions of your metabolism. As Bob Arking, a professor of biology and gerontology at Wayne State University, put it so well, referring to the homeostatic defenses against entropy: "The most fundamental aging process that we can yet identify is the decrease in the organism's ability to repair, maintain, and replace" its molecules, cells, and tissues.[51] In other words, you lose your gardener and the weeds take over.

According to the model of aging proposed by Marion Lamb, an Oxford University zoologist, in her book *The Biology of Ageing*, the first factor in aging involves damage to the cell and its molecules—or entropy. The second is the cell's ability to defend itself against that damage and to repair damage that occurs—its homeostasis. The third factor is the failure of your defenses as you age. Homeostasis becomes less effective at repairing the ravages of entropy. You slowly develop more and more structural and enzymatic abnormalities (Lamb's fourth factor), causing cellular inefficiency (the fifth), and progressive problems in the tissues, organs, and systems of your body (the sixth), culminating finally in your inability to cope with your environment (the seventh and last factor). The unmentioned eighth factor is death.[52]

Lamb is right, but where is the clock that starts the process, allowing your defenses to fail? Each level fails as a result of failure at a more basic level: first the clock, which controls the genes; then gene expression; then the cell's proteins; then the cell; then the tissue; and so on. The clock runs down, genes express a different, senescent pattern, and your defenses fail. Once your defenses are turned down, the process is as inevitable as an avalanche. Damaged proteins and oxidized lipid membranes begin to accumulate. DNA repair and protein transcription slow down, and free radicals increase in concentration. In stately progression, your tissues, organs, and systems slowly and subtly fail, and your clinical decline becomes more obvious every day. Your immune system is not as vigilant or discerning, your kidneys filter less, your lungs lose resilience and capacity, your muscles lose mass and strength, your blood vessels lose elasticity and gain cholesterol, and your brain loses cells and, with it, function. A bump, a push, an increasingly minor stress, and we die.

But what actually shuts off your defenses, shifting the balance to the side of entropy? Whatever it is certainly is the cause of aging. If we can understand this basic mechanism that controls and initiates the cascade of devastation, we will understand aging. And understanding aging may allow us to slow, stop, or reverse its—so far—inevitable course into suffering, sickness, and death.

Only in this century have we begun to acquire the tools to follow aging down to the molecular level where it begins. With the advent of genetics, cell biology, and biochemistry, we are now able to make sense of its mechanisms. Advances in genetic research have given us an understanding of the expression of our genes, which helps us understand not only entropy and homeostasis, but also the mechanism that shifts the balance from your defenses toward entropy. We know that our genes define the limits of those defenses, but we also know that they determine when that bulwark will fail. Your genes contain their own clock that initiates the aging cascade. The clock varies from species to species and individual to individual, paralleling the genetic differences among species and among individuals.

The differences in life span and aging may have lessons for us, in understanding not only how aging works, but the consequences of its being altered.

Aging is universal among many-celled organisms; plants, fungi, and animals all age. But there is a great deal of variability in simpler organisms. Bacteria and viruses don't normally age, for instance, though many other one-celled organisms do. The line is much clearer between germ cells, which do not age, and somatic cells, which do. Although the distinction between somatic and germ cells is uncertain in some organisms,[53] the observation that somatic cells age and germ cells do not is the closest thing we have to a universal rule of aging. Germ cells don't age because they are needed for life to survive. Somatic cells support germ cells, and so have an important function. Then why do they age and die?

There might not be any reason at all. Nature doesn't care about you after you reproduce. Your genes support you until you have reproduced, and have assured your offspring their own chance of reproducing, and after that you are on your own. Evolution has a vested interest in giving you a fair chance of passing on your germ cells, but after that you are of little use. It wants to be sure you become a parent, but then it turns you out into the cold.

But aging is not passive, either, simply "leaving you on your own" after you reproduce. To the contrary, if you might decrease the likelihood of your offsprings' survival, evolution will actively ensure your death. In the Pacific salmon, accelerated aging and death occur within hours after spawning. Whatever the evolutionary reason for that, it isn't a passive process: Aging doesn't just "happen," but is orchestrated and enforced. As we will see in Chapter 4, the clock that sets the aging process in motion may be reset or even turned off, yet evolution goes to a great deal of trouble to ensure that the gene that allows germ cells to be immortal is not only repressed, but *multiply* repressed in the case of somatic cells. That is not passive aging. Aging does not "just happen" because evolution no longer cares. Evolution cares very much: It demands that you age and does so very actively.

Does this prove that aging is actively programmed? Not necessarily. It may be that, in fact, evolution doesn't care whether you age or not, but it *very much* cares about some other goal that is unavoidably linked to the mechanism that causes aging. Suppose, for example, that cancers—including those in young organisms that have not yet reproduced, but are crucial to continuing the species—can only be avoided by a mechanism whose "incidental" side effect was to cause aging in organisms that had already reproduced. Evolution might have no ax to grind regarding your aging after reproduction, but a great deal of interest in preventing cancer, and other life-threatening diseases, in young organisms in order to enable the germ cell line to go on. Such a mechanism would be actively selected for, even if the incidental outcome was aging. Aging is not actively selected for, but the clock itself is.

All of this matters because it tells us something about the difficulty of attempting to reverse aging, and the side effects it will entail. If aging is passive, then we can expect that there is no single mechanism, or even a few mechanisms, that may easily be reversed. On the other hand, if it is passive, then the biological consequences of reversing aging probably won't be great since evolution has no stake in it. In that case, reversing aging will be extremely difficult, but might have few biological repercussions.

But aging isn't passive. Because it is active or incidental, we can expect a narrow set of mechanisms that might easily be reversed or bypassed to allow extended longevity, although we have to wonder about the consequences, to the species and our planet, of altering a mechanism that evolution finds so very important. In the case of incidental aging, the consequences will not be of as much concern as in that of active aging, but whatever the linked mechanism is (cancer, for example) it will be a source of considerable problems for us. As we will also see, that is a problem that we can deal with using the same therapy that will allow us to reverse aging in the first place.

THE TICKING CLOCK

I wasted time, and now doth time waste me;
For now hath time made me his numbering clock;
My thoughts are minutes.

—*RICHARD II*, V.v.

To alter aging, we must find and alter the clock; to find the clock, we must know what it looks like and where to look for it. Alex Comfort, perhaps our most eminent gerontologist, put it clearly in his classic work, *Ageing: The Biology of Senescence*, when he said:

The primary assignment for gerontology—that of finding an accessible mechanism that times the human life-span as we observe it—remains undischarged. But it is nonetheless far closer to that objective today than when we last reviewed the subject—partly because, through the growth of experimental evidence which the pretheories of the past have generated, the possibility of a hierarchy of aging processes integrated by a life-span "clock" has come to be recognized and the nature of that clock is becoming clearer.[54]

What clues do we have that will help us find this clock and how will we identify it correctly when we do find it? Within this century, particularly in the past few decades, most researchers have come to agree that the clock exists. Now we need to identify it. It is as though we were told that a clock was somewhere in our kitchen, but to find it, you need to know what it looks like. Is it a digital or an alarm clock? Is it built into the oven or is it a wristwatch? How big is it and how much does it weigh? What color is it? Is it red, black, or blue? Does it tick or does it hum? What features would be incompatible with the correct clock and what features *must* it have? What are the requirements for our candidates for the aging clock? We already know, in a rough way, where it lies and how it works.

The clock is genetic. All aspects of aging are under genetic control, which means that, although environmental and entropic factors have an impact on aging, it is your genes that ultimately determine—by how well they defend you, or fail to, against environmental effects and entropic damage—the way in which you age. As we age, our genes downregulate, weaken, or turn off our defenses.

Moreover the clock that represses those defenses is the same one that stops cell replication with aging.

Not only does the clock control gene expression and cell division, but it continually rewinds (in the case of germ cells) and then runs down once the germ cell divides and develops into somatic cells.

Nor are germ cells the only ones with a clock that never runs down. Cancer cells also avoid this kind of death. Cancer cells are characterized by two features. First, they pay no attention to cues telling them not to divide and spread, such as hormones or other signals from neighboring cells, and hence they ignore their "duty" to the tissue in which they live. Second, they divide long past their normal Hayflick limit. In cancer cells, as in germ cells, the clock that limits cell replication and that causes repression of homeostatic defenses is either turned off or, as we will see, continuously being reset.

Could the clock that determines aging be the same one that times developmental events in the organism? During growth, the organism's cells must divide in correct sequence and in coordination with other cells—not too early or late. They must express the correct molecules—hormones, growth factors, and chemical signals of myriad functions—at exactly the right moment with respect to the development of distant cells. Certain cells must connect with precise timing in order to function correctly. The entire organism must work as a unit when it is born. It must go through precisely ordered postnatal developmental stages, with behaviors and endocrine levels appropriate for age, allowing for growth, learning, puberty, and reproduction. Could the clock that is responsible for all of this be the same clock that times aging?

It is unlikely. A major feature of aging is the lack of coordination as the organism slowly falls apart. Entropy is given free rein in a stochastic, sloppy manner, not a rigid, precise one. The aging clock is too haphazard and the biochemical sequence of events too unplanned and random to meet the requirements of development. Development is graceful and precise; aging is neither. The developmental clock often uses time units of hours and days to measure and build; the aging clock estimates time in decades to permit destruction and entropy. These are different clocks.

The clock must either tick in all your cells or at least in all of them that age. Its rate must parallel the rate of aging in those cells. Or perhaps not. If we have three cells that age, and only one has a running clock, can the other two take their timing from the one with the running clock? Could the aging of one cell place so heavy a burden on its neighbors that they also show the effects of aging? Could some of the physiological and clinical expression of aging be secondary to neighboring, or even distant, cells? Probably. If a cell is unable to reasonably control production or confinement of free radicals, the cell next to it will likely suffer. If a cell turns over proteins slowly, it might increase the number of damaged protein—or lipid or carbohydrate—molecules around it and cause secondary damage to nearby cells. If the glial cells that surround nerve cells and support them metabolically, age, the nerve cells might be damaged or killed. If the nerve cell "ages," is it the glial cell's fault?

Much of what we call aging is a gross, average clinical outcome: dementia, coronary artery disease, cancer, waning and misdirected immunity. How many of these clinical expressions are the direct result of the cellular dysfunction associated with aging? And how many are the effects of cells that don't really age that much, but are the victims of other cells that do? It may be that the clock—while present in all cells—runs fast in some, slowly in others, and almost not at all in yet others.

What are the characteristics of our clock, then? It must be:

1. part of your genetic library
2. either an active clock or a clock that is crucial for your survival—by preventing cancer, for instance—but incidentally causes aging
3. able to cause a senescent pattern of expression in those genes that are responsible for dealing with free radicals, protein turnover rates, and DNA repair enzymes
4. capable of stopping cell replication after a fixed number of cycles characteristic of the cell
5. stopped, bypassed, or continually reset in germ cells
6. stopped, bypassed, or continually reset in cancer cells
7. unidirectional and able to run down and finally come to a stop

Over the years, a number of candidates for such a mechanism have been offered, including the accumulation of waste products, passive damage to DNA, methylation of DNA, loss of special tissues, and others. However, none of these meets all of the criteria required of an underlying clock for aging. As we will see, in the early 1970s a new suggestion was made for a different kind of clock that might count down and cause aging. It was based on the observation that DNA does not fully duplicate itself in somatic cells. The suggestion languished. Only in the late 1980s was it taken seriously. In 1990, the first paper appeared that not only identified the clock, but supported it strongly with research results.

That clock is the telomere.

CHAPTER 3

THE CLOCK

THE SECOND FATE

The fates . . . Clotho spun the thread of each mortal's life. . . .
Lachesis measured the thread of each mortal's life, thus de-
termining its length. . . . Atropos . . . used her dreaded shears
to cut the thread of each mortal's life.

—ROSENBERG AND BAKER, *MYTHOLOGY AND YOU*

TELOMERES, THE CLOCKS of aging, are the end segments of DNA on chromosomes. Each cell has 46 chromosomes, or 23 chromsome pairs.[1] Each chromosome has two ends, each end with its own telomere, for a total of 92 telomeres per cell. The mature human body has 100 trillion cells, so inside each of us there are 10 quadrillion telomeres.

The telomere is made up of the last several thousand DNA bases as well as the associated proteins that are bound to them, and the telomere is peculiar in several respects. At the end of the telomere the DNA bases do not simply dangle loosely, but form a complex "hairpin" turn with the last several base pairs. We are still not clear about the exact formation of this hairpin, but it appears to be a four-stranded "cloverleaf," called the G-quartet structure (for the guanine bases that it comprises).[2] Also, the telomere is a gene-free region: It does not code for any proteins, even though it plays a critical role in chromosomal function—as do many other gene-free regions of the chromosome.

And, unlike the rest of the chromosome, the sequence of DNA bases in the telomere is invariant and repetitive. In humans (and in all vertebrates) the sequence consists solely of the following repeated bases: thymine, thymine, adenine, guanine, guanine, guanine. Two thymines, an adenine, and three guanines, on every telomere, in every cell, in every one of us. In the telomere, this TTAGGG sequence (or T_2AG_3) is repeated more than a thousand times without any—as yet—observed variation or alteration.

Although the telomeric repeats vary somewhat among different organisms, there is no variety within the vertebrates. Fish, amphibians, reptiles, birds, and mammals all share the same repeated telomere sequence. These organisms diverged from one another more than 400 million years ago, but they retain the identical TTAGGG sequence.[3] The dinosaurs had the same telomere structure that we have today. Vastly different organisms share this sequence, including slime molds, some fungi, and some protozoans (such as the ones that cause sleeping sickness).[4] But even organisms with different telomere sequences do not differ by much. All living things with nuclei also have guanine-rich telomeres and almost all have simple, predictable repeats.

When alteration first occurs as we move down the chromosome away from the end of the telomere, it is subtle, perhaps only a base or two in one of the repeats—small changes in the previously predictable, repetitive pattern. This region of subtly altered sequence is the subtelomeric region, also called the "x region" or "telomere associated DNA."[5] Instead of simple TTAGGG repeats, there might be slight variations, like TAGGG, TTTGGG, TTAAGG, and others.[6] Together, the telomere and the subtelomere make up the "terminal restriction fragment," or TRF, of the chromosome.

Moving farther along toward the middle of the chromosome, and finally out of the subtelomeric region altogether—and therefore out of the terminal restriction fragment—the variability increases until the

DNA sequences become unique and complex, bearing little resemblance to the telomeric repeat sequence (TTAGGG). It is here that your first genes, your "peritelomeric" genes, occur.

If the TTAGGG sequence is so fixed and immutable within the telomere, isn't the exact size known as well? The discussion so far has referred vaguely to "several thousand" repeats. As we will soon see, the telomere's size depends upon one's age, and its relation to aging will be the focus of the rest of this book. But how did we come to understand not only what the telomere is—its size and composition—but what it does and how its length is a key to aging?

HISTORY

Darwin's "survival of the fittest" is really a special case of a more general law of "survival of the stable." The universe is populated by stable things. A stable thing is a collection of atoms that is permanent enough or common enough to deserve a name.

—RICHARD DAWKINS, THE SELFISH GENE

Human interest in aging goes back at least five thousand years, to the ancient time referred to in *The Epic of Gilgamesh*: This is a short time compared with the billions of years that life on our planet has been aging. We have known about the telomere's existence for only slightly more than half a century, and until the last ten years our knowledge of it has been minimal; only in the last five years have we come to see the telomere's connection to aging.

The telomere has survived for more than a billion years. Telomeres have been in cells since they first developed nuclei; prior to that development, their history is unknown. Cells with nuclei and chromosomes protected within those nuclei, eukaryotes, almost all have telomeres.

We know very little about the evolution of the telomere. It may have begun during the early history of life on earth when RNA[7] and not DNA made up the pages of each genetic library, and proteins may have filled some of the same roles that DNA and RNA now fill. In any case, it is likely that the telomere is this old not only because it is so widespread, but also because the telomere is made by an enzyme called telomerase, which is probably a product of that earlier time: Telomerase is not a simple protein—as other enzymes are—but is part protein and part RNA; it is a curious "molecular fossil,"[8] with extremely few parallels in biology.[9]

The word *telomere* was coined by Hans Muller, a biologist, in 1938,[10] fifteen years before James Watson and Francis Crick published their description of the double helix, its base pairing, and the notion that it might provide a mechanism for DNA replication.[11] Based on his work with X-ray damage of chromosomes, Muller already suspected that the telomeres (the word is a combination of the Greek *telos*, meaning "end," and *meros*, "part") capped the ends of the chromosomes and prevented their "fraying" at the exposed ends.

In the 1940s, another biologist, Barbara McClintock, convincingly demonstrated this in her work on maize. She found that without telomeres, chromosomes would break apart and act as though they were "sticky," fusing inappropriately with other chromosomes.[12] Not only would they break up and stick to other chromosomes, but without telomeres they would not separate properly during cell division. It was easy to conclude that telomeres were necessary to chromosomal survival and to cell replication.

The telomere languished somewhat for several decades, until James Watson made a curious observation regarding DNA replication.[13] In 1972, he pointed out that every time a normal, linear chromosome duplicates, it would become shorter, which he called the "end replication problem." To understand how this occurs, a few simple facts about copying DNA strands are necessary. DNA strands can be copied in only one direction. The process is begun by a set of "primers," enzymes that latch on to a single DNA strand in a number of places and begin the copying process. The primer doesn't copy anything, it just primes the enzyme (DNA polymerase) that does real work. The copying enzyme moves on down the DNA strand, copying as it does, while the primer separates, its job now finished. The copying enzyme can only work in one direction on the DNA molecule. It's as though each DNA strand were a one-way street: The primer starts the process and then leaves, letting the copying enzymes continue on down the street.

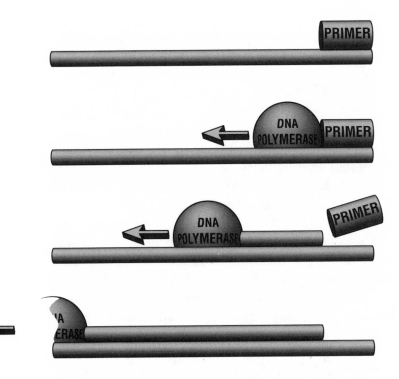

The "end replication problem":
the telomere shortens

Fig. 3.1

Watson pointed out that in each replication of a chromosome, the primer nearest the telomere starts the enzyme copying, but the enzymes can never copy the place where the endmost primer attached itself because they can't go backward, and so, with each replication there will be an area that doesn't get copied and the chromosome will shorten.

In reality, however, it's not one street, but two. Imagine that we have a two-lane highway from East City to West City: Each side of the highway is one way and the sides are separated by an area of grass and trees. Imagine that we are going to "copy" the two sides of the highway by resurfacing them. Look at just one of the sides of the highway. A series of several dozen paving machines (the primers and DNA duplicating enzymes) each start at a different place on the highway and they begin resurfacing (replicating the DNA). As they reach the new pavement already laid down by another paving machine, they finish joining the asphalt surfaces and then leave. The result is a seam-less replication of the highway (the chromosome) from East City to West City.

The problem is that, in our analogy, if no paving machine began exactly in East City, but only a mile outside of it, there will be a mile of highway that never gets resurfaced at the East City end. If the same error occurs each time you resurface the highway, and if each time the crews start a bit farther from East City (farther down on the telomere) a part of the highway will be progressively lost with each resurfacing. In terms of your cells, every time they divide—and the chromosome duplicates—you will lose some pieces of your telomere.

Theoretically, the chromosome should shorten until it disappeared and the process would then continue, destroying our genes once the telomere was gone. Our cells would die, and yet the germ cell line proves that this doesn't happen (at least in germ cells). So either Watson was wrong about shortening chromosomes—he wasn't—or, as he supposed, the chromosome has some mechanism for reextending the missing segments of the telomere. But even before Watson pointed out the problem, a Russian biologist, Alexei Olovnikov had begun to wonder if this shortening served a practical function in biology,[14] that is, if the gradual shortening of the chromosome could act as the clock for cellular aging. His idea was simple and entirely correct.

Unfortunately for Olovnikov—and for most biologists—he wondered about it in Russian. He published his ideas on this subject a year before Watson did, but it was two years before anyone translated his paper into English,[15] and it was not until 1975 that the idea was noticed by Cal Harley—then a graduate student and researcher at McMaster University in Canada—who read the 1973 English version of Olovnikov's paper in the *Journal of Theoretical Biology*. His adviser had gone on sabbatical and Harley presented Olovnikov's paper at a weekly lab meeting on "Theories of Aging" that he'd organized. He and Bob Shmookler Reis began to look at the abundance of repetitious DNA as a function of cellular aging. Although little was known about telomere structure in the mid-1970s, it was clearly composed of repetitive bases, whatever the sequence was. Repetitive DNA sequences decreased with age, but that didn't prove that the repetitions came from the telomere, and it certainly didn't prove that the loss of repetitions caused senescence in cells.

In order to prove that the telomere itself was shortening, as Watson and Olovnikov said it must be, there had to be a way to identify the telomere unambiguously. At about the same time, Liz Blackburn (then at the University of California at Berkeley)—who along with several other researchers was trying to unravel the mystery of the telomere— finally sequenced several telomeres from different species, beginning with a microscopic parameciumlike organism called tetrahymena, that had the advantage of having a lot of telomere to sequence.[16] Over the next few years, several sequences became known: enough to clearly identify the telomere and distinguish it from the rest of the chromosome.

By 1986, Howard Cooke and his group in Edinburgh found that telomeres from somatic cells were clearly shorter than telomeres from germ cells.[17] Yet, as Watson and Olovnikov knew, if somatic cells shorten their telomeres and germ cells do not, germ cells had to have some special mechanism that kept them from shortening or they would have been extinguished long ago.

Did the fact that somatic cells have shorter telomeres than germ cells—as Olovnikov and Watson would have predicted—imply that older cells had shorter telomeres than young cells? And if the germ cell line telomeres didn't shorten, what was the mechanism that corrected the loss of telomeric DNA?

While Cal Harley and his colleagues tried to answer the first of these questions, the second occupied the attention of Carol Greider, a biologist at Cold Spring Harbor Laboratory in New York, who struggled to understand how tetrahymena could keep its telomere from shrinking with every division—as Watson and Olovnikov had said it must. The enzyme responsible was given a name—telomerase—but next to nothing was known about how it worked. As Greider struggled to understand how telomerase worked, she became adept at measuring the telomere, an ability that was about to become crucial to Harley's work.

Harley's attempts to pin down telomere length and aging were initially hampered by not knowing the telomere sequence, but by the late 1980s, the sequence was discovered and he was ready to find out if older cells had shorter telomeres. Fortuitously, Carol Greider and Cal Harley met through a mutual friend and fellow biologist, Bruce Futcher, and the seeds of a fruitful collaboration were sown. Harley wanted to know how the telomere changed with age; Greider had the means to measure it.

Late in the summer of 1988, Greider called Harley to say that Robin Allshire, a colleague of hers at Cold Spring Harbor, had discovered the human telomere sequence and that she and Futcher were ready to measure human telomere lengths. Harley prepared DNA from young and old human fibroblast cultures—and from young and old humans as well—and sent them to Greider without telling her which was which. Greider measured the telomeres and called him with the results: It was apparent that young telomeres were longer than old ones—consistently. The length of their telomeres clearly identified the number of times the cells had divided in culture (or in the body), how many generations had passed, and how close they were to their Hayflick limit when cellular aging would shut them down. For the first time, telomere length was shown to be related to aging in cells. Similar results in other cells soon followed their work.[18]

At conception, your telomere is about 10,000 base pairs long, and by birth it has already shortened to about 5,000 base pairs, or about 800 TTAGGG repeats. The subtelomeric region is approximately another 5,000 base pairs long, and here the TTAGGG sequence becomes increasingly random. Together these two regions—the telomere plus the subtelomere that together form the terminal restriction fragment—are about 15,000 base pairs long at conception, about 10,000 base pairs long at birth. Compared with the rest of the chromosome and its genes, the telomere is relatively small. An average chromosome is 130,000,000 base pairs long, or about 25,000 times as long as the human telomere at birth. The average gene is about 120,000 base pairs long, or about 25 times the length of the human telomere at birth.

In a seminal paper in *Nature* in 1990, Harley, Greider, and Futcher published their results and resurrected Olovnikov's and Watson's idea of the telomere as the clock for cellular aging, and perhaps for aging in the organism itself. Ironically, publication was delayed because one of *Nature*'s editors twice rebutted the paper, questioning how the data could be so remarkable. It was difficult to accept an idea that was so simple and elegant. But finally it was published, probably due to the backing of James Watson.

The paper in *Nature* was not the end of the story; rather, it was the beginning. Our story now shifts, first to an exploration of the telomere itself, and then to a consideration of how telomere shortening affects cancer, aging, and the reversal of the aging process. The telomere determines not only the aging of the cell, but much more: what diseases we contract and which ones we die of, at what rate and in what ways we age.

THE TIME COMES

"The time has come," the walrus said, "to talk of many things."

—LEWIS CARROLL, "THE WALRUS AND THE CARPENTER"

In addition to serving as a clock for aging, the telomere has a multitude of other functions, among them these four main ones:[19]

1. Protecting the end of the chromosome from damage or faulty recombination
2. Allowing complete replication of the chromosome
3. Controlling gene expression
4. Aiding in organizing the nuclear chromosomes

Until recently, these four functions have been the focus of most telomere research. They are of concern to us because they may be the reason that the telomere acts as an aging clock at all. The repeating bases of the telomere and the protein structure at the end of the chromosome have evolved for more important reasons to the organism than aging. Aging may be just an incidental, but inseparable, effect of critical cellular needs that can only be met by the telomeric structure.

These four telomere functions can be divided into two broad categories. The first two functions are necessary for flawless inheritance of genetic information; they allow the organisms to reproduce. The second two allow the cell access to the genes in a controlled and efficient manner; they allow the organisms to survive. The first function, protection of the end of the chromosome, is the most universally agreed upon and the one that was identified earliest. Chromosomes without "caps" break apart and fuse with other chromosomes. As the chromosome breaks apart, it may divide a gene; as it fuses with another chromosome, it may weld together two unrelated genes. Either action risks destroying genetic information by disrupting the normal base sequence of a gene: Either may be fatal to the cell or to the organism that inherits such damaged genes.

The second function of the telomere—to allow replication of the chromosome—is also essential to genetic inheritance. Each time the cell replicates its chromosomes, a small piece of DNA is taken off the end of each chromosome. It appears that the telomere's long, repetitive TTAGGGs are meant to be lost; they provide a buffer against the constant, and unavoidable, loss of bases during replication.

While this is necessary to your somatic cells, your germ cells go them one better by reextending the buffer. A special enzyme, telomerase reextends the telomere (adding TTAGGGs) as the loss occurs.[20] Surprisingly, and with remarkably few exceptions, only germ cells respond to this constant erosion during replication by reextending their telomeres.

This same second function of the telomere—protection against chromosomal erosion and gene loss—is dealt with very differently in some organisms. Instead of having a telomere at all, they form ring chromosomes (without any ends to lose pieces from) or "hairpins" (which can replicate "around the corner"). For example, some bacteria do the former; pox viruses, such as smallpox and chicken pox, do the latter.

Why are the telomeres made up of TTAGGGs? Is this set of bases the only one that can buffer against erosion? No; there are a number of other sequences, although for some reason they almost universally have a large number of Gs—guanines—in them. Is there something special about this particular base that is needed to fulfill the second function of the telomere? Perhaps. We know that the guanines form a "knot" on the end of the telomere. The presence of this structure may prevent degradation of the end of the chromosome when the cell is not replicating, just as the telomere buffers against loss when it is.[21]

The third function of the telomere is to control genes near the end of the chromosome. Our research has yet to show us how this works and all we know is that some species use telomeres for this function, and perhaps they all do. When it is used, the telomere regulates the genes adjacent to the telomere (peritelomeric genes).[22] It is likely that proteins bound to the telomere exert a "downstream" effect on the peritelomeric genes. Altering the expression of these critical genes may play a central role in aging: As the telomere shortens, gene expression alters.

The fourth function is to aid in organizing the books in your genetic library. This hypothetical function has two parts: organization during cell division (when your books are packed into boxes and are ready to move into a newly divided cell), and organization between divisions (when you are actually using your library books for reference). Either of these is likely to occur in some—perhaps all—species. The telomere might provide one of the physical "handles" that the cell can use to move the books to the daughter cell. Or when the cell is using the books, telomeres may help in organizing the chromosomes, forming handles that resemble "bouquets," a poetic, but accurate description.[23] Considering the size of your library books (relative to the sentences you must access regularly and rapidly), it may be crucial to have an organizer that prevents the book from becoming jumbled. However, we still do not know whether either of these putative organizational functions is actually used in the human cell.[24]

Does the telomere do anything else? Yes. It has a few other possible functions and one other major function. The telomere may be an initiation site for the matching of homologous chromosomes, moving analogous genes from one chromosome to another prior to dividing them up among daughter cells. The fact that similar TTAGGGs are scattered along the length of the chromosome and are probably attachment sites for this recombination suggest that the telomere is probably an attachment site as well.[25] As we come to know more about this surprisingly important section of the chromosome, some of these functions will turn out to be unrelated to the telomere; others will become apparent and surprise us.

There is, of course, a fifth function of the telomere that is becoming readily apparent and has already surprised us. The telomere functions as a clock that regulates aging.

THE CLOCK UNWINDS

Till like a clock worn out with eating time,
The wheels of weary life at last stood still.

—JOHN DRYDEN

OVERVIEW

The telomeric clock is elegantly simple, yet at the same time is extraordinarily complex. This chapter presents the aging mechanisms—along with some of their complexity—while providing an appreciation of the telomere's simplicity as the unifying, underlying timer for cellular and, in the end, organismal aging. This section is divided into several subsections, each of which addresses a basic question about the telomeric clock.

The first question concerns the linkage between the shortening of the telomere and the suppression of genes that are responsible for basic cell functions, and how this controls the cell cycle. Linkage of the telomere to gene expression can affect the cell in two ways: gradually and cumulatively over the life of a cell lineage, or in a relatively sudden, all-or-nothing fashion when a telomere "runs out" of TTAGGG repeats. We will review the cell cycle, discussing how a cell decides whether or not to divide, and how the cell avoids cancer—and division—when its DNA is damaged.

The second question involves *when* this gradual loss of telomeric repeats begins to stop the cell cycle and affect gene expression. Telomeric repeats are not simply lost in a predictable, evenly paced fashion. The loss varies among telomeres within a cell and varies among cells, even ones that are otherwise identical.

How short does a telomere have to be to cause cellular aging? And which telomere causes it? For cellular aging to occur, do all ninety-two telomeres have to go? Why does the cell have ninety-two telomeric clocks? How do those clocks coordinate, if they coordinate at all?

Telomere lengths differ among different chromosomes in any cell;

they differ among cells, tissues, and organs. How do these differences in telomere lengths determine when aging occurs?

If our first two questions concern the relationship of telomere shortening, and its variability, to the cell, the third extends those questions: How do the processes of telomere shortening, gene repression, and aging in one cell relate to its neighboring cells that make up a tissue, an organ, or the whole organism? A cell is rarely independent of other cells. So how does one cell's telomere affect another? The cell is a part of a "society": a tissue, an organ, an organism. It has duties to its neighboring cells. As a cell ages, it alters and often forgoes those duties, and, as a result, neighboring cells—and hence tissues and organs—become dysfunctional. The neighboring cells show aging changes. The result is aging of the organism and an increasing likelihood of death.

And finally, how does the telomeric clock fit into the overall discussion of aging and its reversal?

HOW THE TELOMERE AFFECTS GENES

Gene Regulation

As gene expression changes with age, the cell makes more of some proteins and less of others. Since everything the cell does is based on proteins, as the protein production changes so do cell functions. Certain proteins—such as EF-1, which is critical to the production of other proteins—become scarce and protein turnover declines throughout the cell. Regulation of cell division, a special case of gene regulation, strikes to the heart of both aging and cancer. In old age, the cells often stop dividing when they should keep dividing. In cancer, the cells continue dividing when they should stop. In both cases, regulation of cell division, among other things, has failed and the organism fails and dies.

There are two prongs to the linkage between telomere shortening and gene regulation: The first involves the changes that occur in the "hood" covering the telomere as the telomere shortens, and the second involves the effects on gene expression when the TTAGGG repeats are entirely used up. Either of these mechanisms can increase or decrease gene expression—quite likely simultaneously activating some genes and repressing others. But both alter the expression of genes.

Hood Changes

Properly defined, the telomere is the entire structure at the end of the chromosome, not just the repeating TTAGGGs. It not only includes this DNA, but also the proteins, and RNA, that are closely attached to the TTAGGGs, and which control gene expression. Those proteins bind to the chromosome and give it one of two distinct appearances. It can be thin and elongated, a form called euchromatin ("true chromatin"); in that form, the genes are relatively exposed and more likely to be expressed. Or the chromosome can be short and bunched, a form called heterochromatin ("other chromatin"); in that form, the genes are less exposed, and less likely to be expressed.

Normally, the telomere's hood covers not only the telomere, but also the subtelomere and a good portion of the peritelomeric genes. By covering the genes, it restricts gene expression in the peritelomeric region in many, if not all, species.[26] As the telomere shortens, the hood changes, forcing gene expression to change as well. Generally, the hood appears to shrink as the telomere shortens, as though the telomere was less able to maintain as large a hood. So as the telomere shortens, the heterochromatin hood is less tightly bound and it shortens, exposing the activating peritelomeric genes, previously covered up and sup-

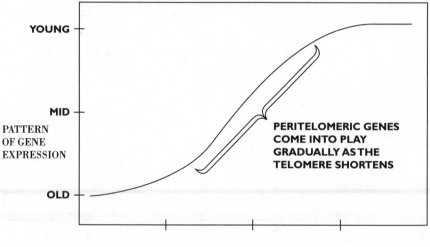

YOUNG

MID

PATTERN
OF GENE
EXPRESSION

OLD

PERITELOMERIC GENES
COME INTO PLAY
GRADUALLY AS THE
TELOMERE SHORTENS

TELOMERE LENGTH

Fig. 3.2

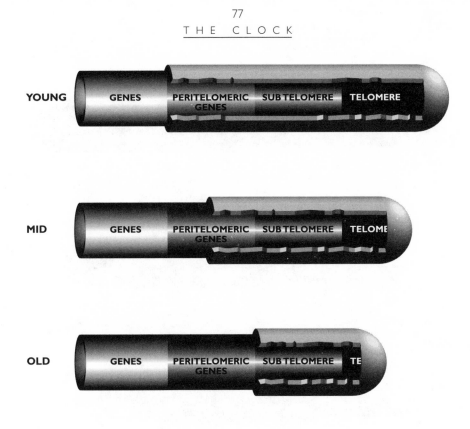

THE SHRINKING HOOD

Fig. 3.3

pressed by the hood. Those genes, in turn, begin producing proteins that suppress other genes.

Although it is likely that the hood shrinks in humans, it is possible that in some species, the hood might not shrink as the telomere shortens,[27] but might remain the same size and slide downward on the chromosome, covering more peritelomeric genes, rather than uncovering them. That could occur if the heterochromatin hood size was independent of telomere size and the telomere served only to anchor it at its most distant end.

Altering gene expression is the heart of aging in a cell. Genes that make crucial enzymes, such as the elongation factor one (EF-1), are suppressed. That enzyme is responsible for lengthening most proteins as they are made; since you make less as cells age, the production rate for many proteins falls. The same is true of dozens of other enzymes, such as catalase, which is partly responsible for holding free radicals at bay. As fewer proteins are produced, the turnover rate falls. Mitochon-

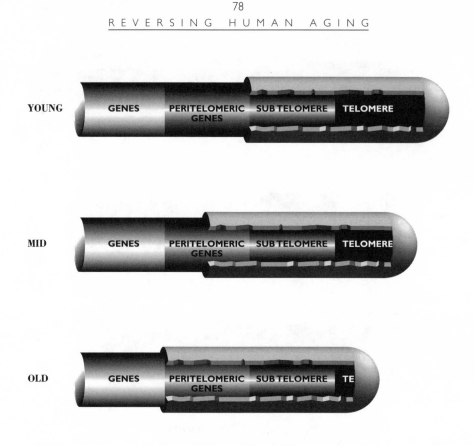

THE SLIDING HOOD

Fig. 3.4

drial membranes grow leakier. DNA repair becomes slower, production of proteins for export decreases, and the cell becomes less and less capable.

Whether the hood shrinks or slides, the end result is the same: Expression of some genes may increase and others decrease as the telomere shortens and regulatory genes are turned on or off. And in either case, the effects on gene expression are gradual and cumulative. Although this appears to mirror, and perhaps explain, the changes that occur as the organism ages, the story is a bit more complex, involving a more unexpected, useful, and remarkable mechanism.

End-Telomere Changes

The changes that result from the end-telomere mechanism are more abrupt than those from the hood. And they may be far more important to the process of aging. They certainly are more important in enhancing our understanding of cancer and cell division.

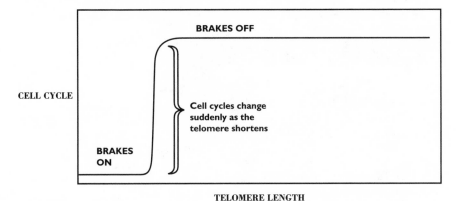

Fig. 3.5

The outline of the mechanism is simple. The cell constantly checks the chromosomes for damage, to determine whether it needs to repair damaged DNA before replicating. Damaged DNA and chromosomes without a telomere are "sticky": Not only do they stick to other broken pieces, but they also bind to special proteins whose only purpose is to signal that such damage has occurred. These "damaged DNA binding proteins," or DDBPs, function as protein monitors to prevent the cell from passing on genetic errors. Binding increases quickly as the telomere reaches its last 1,000 to 500 base pairs. Prior to this point, there is probably almost no binding; by the time the last few hundred TTAGGGs are exposed, the DDBPs are binding fully to the end of the chromosome.

What happens then? When these DDBPs begin congregating on the damaged chromosome, they become unavailable to the rest of the cell. As a result, several other proteins (see Figure 3.6), which are normally held in check by the DDBPs, are released from their restraints. This menagerie of regulatory proteins (p53, Rb, CDK2, Cyclin E, p21, and others) are part of a cascade that prevent the cell from any further division. They do that by turning up the production of a protein that blocks the cell cycle: The cell no longer enters the phase of its cycle in which it copies its chromosomes.[28] And that prevents the cell from replicating the damaged DNA (or shortened telomere) that applied the brake in the first place.

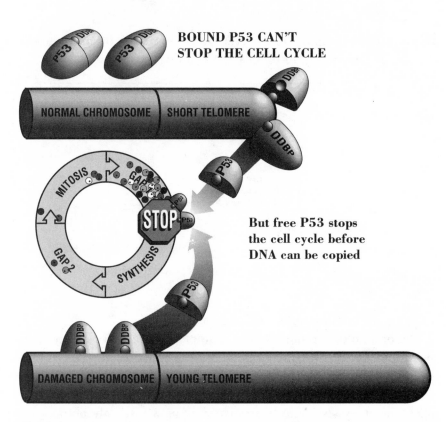

Fig. 3.6

Let's look at this process in greater detail. Each cell has a normal and predictable replication cycle. The first phase is the "first gap," or "G1," phase, so called because it lies between two more active phases: synthesis and mitosis. At the end of the G1 phase, there is a checkpoint at which the cell tests to see if everything is ready to move on to the next phase. If the cell fails any test, the countdown is put on hold until the problems are fixed, if they can be. If the cell passes this first checkpoint (called the G1/S checkpoint), it moves into the S (for synthesis) phase. There, the cell copies its chromosomes. It then enters a second gap phase (G2) followed by the mitosis (M) phase, in which it divides into two daughter cells.

Whether the checkpoints are passed depends on a number of signals; some act like a car's gas pedal, some like the brakes. The G1/S checkpoint—between the first gap phase and the synthesis phase—is the most important one. It responds not only to damaged DNA (which puts on the brakes), but also to signals from other cells acting as either brakes or accelerators, depending on what the body needs. For example, if more red blood cells are needed, a strongly positive signal (stepping on the "gas") is sent to the stem cell that produces your red blood cells, encouraging it to pass G1/S and divide to provide more red blood cells. Skin cells, white blood cells, endothelial cells in the blood vessel walls, and cells that line the gastrointestinal tract all have signals like these that tell them whether or not to divide.

Every cell receives a constant stream of signals from other cells, some prompting it to accelerate (i.e., divide), some to brake. Some of these signals are hormones or metabolic products in the bloodstream, while others derive from direct contact with neighboring cells. All of these signals together—whether instructing the cells to stop or go— determine whether or not a cell should pass the G1/S checkpoint. If it does so, it is then committed to passing the remaining checkpoints;[29] thus the G1/S checkpoint is the pivot for cellular aging and cancer.

If the "brakes" are applied because of DNA damage, but they don't work and the cell divides anyway, the daughter cells will inherit the damage and—if they don't die—may continue to divide. These cells with brakes that have failed are precancerous. Although most will finally die as they reach their Hayflick limits, one in every three million goes on to express telomerase—despite several repressors whose only role is to prevent the telomerase gene from being expressed—becoming a true cancer cell.[30]

It is not clear how cancer cells manage to reexpress telomerase, but the result is plain. The, now reextended, telomere no longer binds DDBPs and the cell is again able to divide as it did when it was younger, allowing continuous and malignant cell division as long as the cancer cell expresses telomerase. Anything that could inhibit telomerase should also prevent the cancer cell from dividing and the tumor from growing, thus eliminating cancer.[31]

Several tumors caused by viruses bypass the G1/S checkpoint by directly inactivating the brakes. Papilloma virus, for example, inactivates the two most important "braking" proteins, p53 and Rb, by producing proteins that are made especially to attach to them (E6 and E7, respectively) and allow cell division to continue unchecked. The same occurs with one of the most infamous "transforming" viruses, SV40, which produces an inactivator called Tag. Tag disconnects the cell's brakes, although the cell still has to express telomerase in order to divide indefinitely. Cancers—whether caused by viruses, toxins, or high-energy photons—all have to express telomerase to survive for long. Not only does the occurrence of malignancies increase as you grow older, but this same braking system is at the heart of the end-telomeric mechanism of aging. As the telomere comes to an end, it is identified as damaged DNA, and the cell slowly brakes to a halt. The telomere provides a buffer against gene loss and damage; the incidental cost, however, is aging.

An aging cell receives two kinds of signals: those from other cells telling it to divide and replace lost cells, and those from its own telomeres revealing that its chromosomes are damaged, or are too short, and that the cell should not replicate its DNA. Until the chromosomes can be repaired, the cell has to wait. But as aging occurs, the chromosome can no longer be repaired; the telomere has worn away. The only way the cell can "fix" the telomere is to express telomerase, but it can't. So the gas pedal and the brake are on simultaneously, which is part of the reason for the altered pattern of gene expression in old cells.

Until the point when it is almost gone, the length of the telomere may be irrelevant; short telomeres can still stabilize chromosomes. But is their pattern of gene expression different? Does it change gradually long before the telomere is gone? The effects on gene expression might be imperceptible until there is one critically short telomere, which is recognized by the checkpoint, stopping the cell cycle. An "SOS" goes out to the cell, as the cell attempts to find and repair the damaged DNA. Unfortunately, telomere repair almost never occurs and the cell finally dies without further division. The telomere functions like a clock; but it is also a genetic time bomb, ticking slowly and innocently until it detonates, bringing the cell to a complete stop.

TELOMERE CHANGES

Telomere Lengths

As a fertilized egg, humans begin life with about 10 kb (10,000 bases) of pure TTAGGG, or perhaps a bit less. That is the extent of your clock. Just downstream from the telomere—in the subtelomeric region—there are probably around 5 kb or so, for a total of about 15 kb of nongenetic bases on each chromosome end. This segment, the terminal restriction fragment (TRF) of the chromosome—telomere and subtelomere—is at its maximum length in the fertilized egg; from that point on, the telomere shrinks with each cell division.[32]

In fact, by the time you are born, there have been enough divisions in an average cell to deplete about half of the ten thousand bases each telomere started with. The length of your terminal restriction fragment has already decreased from 15,000 bases (5,000 in the subtelomere and 10,000 in the telomere) down to 10,000 (5,000 in the subtelomere and only 5,000 in the telomere). You lost 5,000 bases of your telomeric DNA and have only another 5,000 left. You invested half (5,000 of the 10,000 you started with) of your telomere in creating a body at all. By the time you have reached old age, your subtelomeric region may still be as long as 5 kb, but the telomere may be less than 2 kb long. And that is only an average. Telomere length varies not only among individuals and different cells in the same individual, but among different telomeres within a single cell.

Generally, length of the telomere depends on the number of cell divisions the organism has undergone. Cells divide in the fetus; that is how the fertilized egg differentiates and grows, finally becoming you. After birth, telomere shortening loosely parallels the age of the organism, but depends on the cell. These differences in telomere length determine how we age: Some cells divide continuously throughout your life, some cease dividing and maintain themselves for decades in this quiet state, and still others do roughly the same thing, but with the right provocation begin dividing.

The cells that line the gastrointestinal tract, and the ones that form your red blood cells, divide more or less continuously throughout your life. Even in these cell lines, however, the division is carefully orchestrated according to the body's needs: Almost never do the cells divide too often or too seldom; almost never are there too many or too few cells to do the job required of them. The telomeres of your skin fibroblasts shorten continuously throughout your life span, correlating well with your age and even more strongly with how your body has been used. As George Burns put it, "It's not the years, it's the miles."

On the other hand, neurons in the brain—but not the glial cells that surround and support them—divide only in the fetus and usually are incapable of division after birth.[33] They have already undergone myriad divisions from fertilized egg to fully mature and functional nerve cells. Their telomeres shorten in an early prodigality and then stop forever. Roughly, their telomeres are half the length that they were at conception. Their clocks have run down halfway and remain that way—half wound—regardless of your life span, living a cloistered and celibate existence.

Other cells, like liver and immune system cells, divide occasionally and then only when circumstances demand it. Their telomeres vary in length depending on the type of cell, the age of the organism, and the demands life places on them. White blood cells are a good example. The telomeres of white blood cells in an AIDS patient—who has been losing and replacing as many as 1 billion to 2 billion white blood cells per day in the fight—are likely to be shorter than in patients not infected because those cells have been multiplying almost continuously in a fruitless attempt to keep up with their loss to the virus.[34]

Cells that divide continuously may still have perhaps 2 kb left in old age, but that is only an average. One telomere may be long, while the next may be gone entirely. In an aging cell, there is at least one telomere that has lost most of its TTAGGGs. That one telomere is not only enough, it is one too many.

Why Aging Is Gradual

Telomeres come to an abrupt end, but youth does not. We see aging as a slow, cumulative, almost undetectably slow degradation of function over the decades. This process should be explained by a similar gradual mechanism, such as the shift in the heterochromatin hood. How, then, can the end-telomere mechanism, with its abrupt turning off of the cell, explain most of the gradual process of aging?

The first part of the answer might be telomerase expression. If small amounts of telomerase were expressed from time to time, the balance between loss and replacement of TTAGGGs would fluctuate. When the telomere was short, the cell would act old, but if the cell expressed a trace amount of telomerase, the telomere would fluctuate to a length slightly above the cutoff, the cell cycle would begin again, and the cell would act young. Fluctuation near the cutoff (a three-step-forward-two-backward situation) would create the impression, from the gross perspective, that the cell's aging was gradual. Although there is such a near balance between telomerase expression and telomere loss in tumor cells,[35] most normal somatic cells never express telomerase.[36]

The second explanation is that the end-telomere response is not abrupt—at least initially—but is actually graded. The mechanism isn't operative at all when the telomere still has more than a 1,000 base pairs, but comes into play when they fall below that number. At first, the mechanism is sporadic and gradual. The aging response of a cell is graded over the last 500–1,000 base pairs of TTAGGG and only becomes reliable and emphatic as the telomere comes to an end.

The third explanation is that your telomeres recombine. A single short telomere may trigger cellular aging, but a shuffling of the telomeres can occur, stealing pieces from a long one to add length to the shorter one. Robbing Peter to pay Paul may not change the average telomere length, but may save the cell.

Both graded response and recombination are likely to play a role in aging, while the first mechanism, trace telomerase expression, is not. Whatever the mechanisms, the aging cell does not suddenly stop dividing; first it slows considerably. Cell aging is graded over the last several—perhaps a dozen or more—divisions. The brake is first applied gently, then—at the very last—firmly and irrevocably. And even if aging *were* abrupt within the cell, we would still perceive it as gradual. A tissue composed of millions of cells declines gradually, even if individual cells—one by one—aged abruptly. Clinical aging results from overall, gradual loss of telomere length and an overall, gradual loss of function in our cells.

Telomere Variance

Telomere shrinkage alone explains much of cell aging, but a great deal of the aging mechanism, especially the clinical characteristics, depends on the variability in the lengths of the telomeres. Telomere lengths vary both within cells (comparing different telomeres in a single cell) and between cells (comparing average telomere lengths between two cells) and the variance changes with age.[37]

There are several reasons for the variance within cells. As James Watson and Alexei Olovnikov pointed out originally, every time the chromosome is replicated one of the two strands must shorten. That automatically suggests a mechanism for variance. One cell will inherit a short strand, the other a long strand. At the next generation, two cells will have slightly short strands, one an even shorter strand, and one a strand that is still the original length. Theoretically, this process will continue until we have an enormous collection of cells—one with no telomere (on that particular chromosome), one with a telomere with the original number of repeats, and a huge number of cells of any possible length in between. A graph of the telomere lengths of these cells (Figure 3.7) shows a normal bell curve. As you age, more and more cells run up against the zero-bases wall until the organism dies.

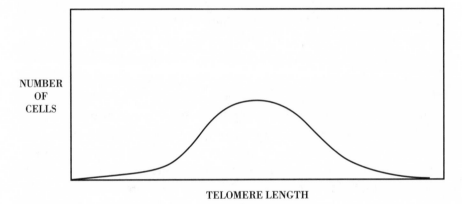

NUMBER
OF
CELLS

TELOMERE LENGTH

Fig. 3.7

Or they would, were if not for the recombination (shuffling) of the chromosomes discussed above.[38] As a result, the likelihood of one cell keeping its long telomere intact over several generations approaches zero. And it is similarly unlikely that a short telomere can be maintained with every division. Telomere shortening is spread around the chromosomes randomly.

Variation is also found in the number of bases lost during replication which is determined by several factors, among them where the DNA polymerase attaches itself to the telomere during replication. Because the distance from the actual end of the telomere varies, the number of bases lost will vary unpredictably from division to division.

Additionally, though the average length of a telomere is 10,000 base pairs at conception, that is only an average, derived from ninety-two telomeres each with slightly different lengths. If a telomere began with only two TTAGGGs, after a few generations variance would be small. (In fact, such a cell probably wouldn't survive long enough for us to measure it at all.) On the other hand, a telomere that begins with hundreds of repeats has enough repeats—and time—to develop a great deal of measurable variance. The longest telomeres are found in germ cells. They don't begin with some uniform, exact length, but vary from one telomere to the next. As far as we know, telomerase doesn't "set" the telomere to any specific length.[39] The length of the telomere in the germ cell line is a product of the rate of TTAGGG loss and the rate of replacement of TTAGGGs by telomerase, both of which vary.

Finally, because of variation in hood lengths, gene expression may vary even if two different chromosomes have exactly the same telomere lengths.

The variability of telomere length among cells is even greater than it is within cells. Cells found in the same tissue—even if they have undergone the same number of divisions—are unlikely to have the same number of telomeric bases because of the many sources of variance within a cell. And having the same average telomere length still doesn't guarantee the same gene expression and degree of aging. In Figure 3.8, the telomeres of both cells have the same average length (5,000 base pairs), but the variation in one is much greater than in the other. The first cell has a range of telomere lengths of 0–10,000 base pairs; the second, of only 4,000–6,000. The result is that the checkpoint

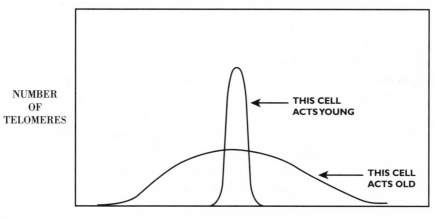

Telomere variance can determine cell "age"

Fig. 3.8

in the first cell detects perhaps a single short telomere and stops cell division, while the second cell continues dividing normally.

But if variability contributes to aging, why should we find that in a group of cells, variance decreases as cells age? If we look at a large group of cells, the variance is initially high; as the group ages, all telomeres—on the average—shorten. Those cells in which the telomere has shortened to a critical length stop dividing, and the telomere doesn't shorten any farther. These cells quietly wait, while others continue shortening their telomeres until they too reach the same critical length.

It is as though the cells were children moving about in a room in which you sat in one corner. Every time one comes within reach, you stop them and make them sit at your feet. As the game continues, the average position of the children becomes closer and their variability drops dramatically because those at your feet don't move about at all. As telomeres age, they too sit quietly, more and more short ones congregating until most of them are short and stubby. When that happens, their variability will also be minimal.

As the telomeres shorten with each division, their cells slow down, until they finally cease to divide and merely mark time, while those with longer telomeres continue to divide and their telomeres shorten. The cells in a "middle-aged" culture have a broad spectrum of telomeres represented; the cells of "old" cultures have a more uniform set of short telomeres. When the telomeres of aging cells are measured in cultures, they exhibit less variability.[40]

The fact that the variance is so great allows us to answer a surprisingly important, but superficially whimsical, question: If the telomere is a clock, then why do you have 92 of them in each of your cells? You don't *need* 92 clocks; but the fact that there are so many of them explains why you age gradually instead of abruptly. The reason that you don't wake up one morning old, gray, wrinkled, and confused is that you have more than a 100 trillion cells and each of them has 92 clocks and that none of these 10 quadrillion clocks keeps exactly the same time.

TISSUES AND ORGANS

The aging of individual cells, and of groups of cells, such as an organ, are related, yet remarkably different: The difference is—occa-

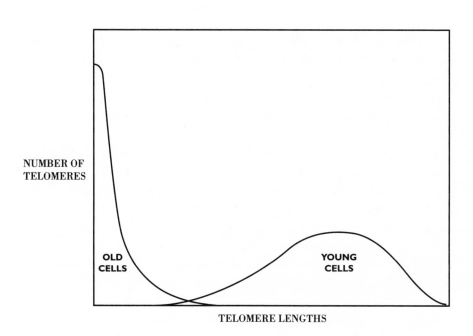

**NUMBER OF
TELOMERES**

**OLD
CELLS**

**YOUNG
CELLS**

TELOMERE LENGTHS

Old telomeres don't vary much

Fig. 3.9

sionally—a matter of life or death. Cell immortality is irrelevant to human life: You can't construct a body out of cancer cells, which are immortal, but lack the cooperative "social" behavior that defines multi-cellular organisms like ourselves. Cellular immortality is not enough to prevent aging.

Cell death, on the other hand, is necessary to your survival. You lose millions, sometimes billions, of skin, intestinal, and blood cells daily so that the remainder of your 100 trillion cells can survive. But you could not survive the loss of the stem cells from which these other cells derive; stem cells replace transient cells such as blood and skin cells. If all your cells died, you would, too; but if all your cells lived, you would still die. And all of these dying and living cells must be coordinated and programmed.

For example, in prenatal development, cells that are no longer neces-sary—the webbing between your fetal fingers, for example—are ordered to die. This intentional homicide is called apoptosis: The cell that receives the fatal signal turns itself off, breaks up, and finally ruptures and dies. In a less dramatic fashion, all of your cells depend upon signals from other cells. Every cell depends upon its neighbors and more distant cells.[41] That coordination is an integral part of the process of aging.

In the same way that cells age from internal cues (from the telomere clock, for instance) or can die as a result of external signals (as in programmed cell death), they also suffer at the hands of external events—such as trauma, infection, and inflammation. As a cell reaches the end of its telomere clock and the cell cycle slows and finally halts, the cell sends out SOS messages that reach neighboring cells. Those signals trigger a multitude of responses: They cause the release of inflammatory substances, such as cytokines, and attract inflammatory cells, such as macrophages, which works to the detriment and even destruction of the cell that sent out the signal; but the cell's neighbors suffer as well. This is part of how many diseases of old age, including osteoarthritis, dementia, and arterial disease, originate.

In addition, as the cell nears the end of its telomeres, it also stops responding correctly to the needs of other cells, causing the neighboring cells to fail as well. But this is not limited to merely neighboring cells. As cells lining your vessels fail, they attract inflammatory cells (macrophages) and build plaques that obstruct the vessel, or the vessel may balloon outward and rupture. As cell function is lost, you lose tissues that depend on the aging vessel. Cells lining the arteries that supply blood to your heart are stressed from high blood sugars, hypertension, and a host of other more minor insults. They divide and replace lost cells, but as their telomeres come to an end, cells are no longer replaced, inflammation occurs, cholesterol plaques are laid down, the artery narrows, and heart muscle dies—and occasionally its owner as well. It begins in a cell, the cumulative effect is local, but the end result widespread and catastrophic.

SUMMARY

As cells cycle and divide, the chromosomes show a random, gradual, but almost unavoidable shortening of their telomeres. Even in the rare somatic cell that expresses small amounts of telomerase, the shortening only slows, but does not stop.

Even as the average length falls, the variation in telomere lengths is initially large. That means that although the damaged DNA binding proteins are more likely to bind, the actual response of the cell is variable and unpredictable. The unpredictability will be even worse among different cells in a given tissue, especially because some will have divided more than others and others will have finished dividing and their telomeres will not be shortening at all. The variability among different tissues and organs will be even greater. The higher you look in the organization of the organism, the more variability you will find and the less predictable will be the specific aging change.

Aging will vary increasingly as we ascend from genes to cells, from cells to tissues, from tissues to organs, and finally—and especially— from organs to the whole body. Not only will it vary in rate of onset and progression, but it will vary unavoidably in expression. Aging is chaotic and ever changing; it expresses itself with endless variety, although the general themes remain the same.

Aging changes are greatest in cells that continue to divide, but are not limited to those cells. Nondividing cells show problems—which we associate with aging—as the cells around them age and cause secondary problems in these otherwise healthy cells. Glial cells age; neurons suffer the consequences. Cells lining the vessels age; the vessels accumulate plaque, and heart muscle—in which the telomeres remain unaltered—dies.

The telomere is the major factor in cellular aging, and cellular aging is the major factor in the body's aging. Most of the body's aging process is a result of the cumulative aging of different cell groups. The aging of your tissues and organs results from the interplay of separate cell groups that no longer respond correctly to cues from other cells.

We have now considered what aging is (in Chapter 2) and what causes it (in this chapter). Aging results from the shortening of telomeres and the variability in their lengths. The cells can no longer divide and they alter their gene expression. Aging cells damage cells around them because the former cannot meet the responsibilities they have to the latter; worse yet, they actively damage those other cells by inflammation and other mechanisms. These cumulative problems affect the function of tissues, organs, and ultimately, the entire body.

But how do we know that the telomere is the stone that starts this avalanche of aging? How do we know that the gradual shortening of the telomere causes aging in the cell, the tissue, or the organism?

CHAPTER 4

WHAT WE KNOW

A T R O U T I N T H E M I L K

Some circumstantial evidence is very strong,
as when you find a trout in the milk.

—HENRY DAVID THOREAU, *WALDEN*

REVERSING AGING

THE KEY TO aging first became clear in 1990, when Cal Harley, Bruce Futcher, and Carol Greider linked the telomere to aging. Since then, we have begun to understand more and more of how the process works—in cells in culture, in other animals, and in humans. But are we right? If we succeed in reversing aging in an old person or preventing it in a young one, then we will know we have understood the process.

First, when we can totally *prevent* aging, we still won't be able to *reverse* all of it, as we will see in considerable detail in Chapter 7. Those elderly who are treated can expect dramatic, rapid results, but not complete reversal of certain aspects of aging. Some things, once broken, cannot be fixed; reversal of aging will only be partial.

Second, although we will soon be able to prevent aging, it will take decades to prove it in humans. It takes so long for us to age that the effects will not be apparent quickly in those who elect to take longevity therapy as young adults. Prevention of aging may be complete, but it will be slow. The ultimate proof of our ability to reverse aging will be in our doing it, not in our theorizing about why we should be able to do it.

Arguments that aging cannot be reversed have been, to date, founded on fact. Except in cells in the laboratory, aging has never yet been reversed.

What is the evidence that we can reverse the aging process?

TALKING CELLS

"Oh, Tiger Lily," said Alice, addressing herself to one that was waving gracefully about in the wind, "I wish you could talk!"

—LEWIS CARROLL, *THROUGH THE LOOKING GLASS*

Tiger lilies, even without speaking, can tell us quite a lot. They can tell us about how fast they grow and age, what soil they like, whether they prefer sun or shade. The best way to obtain certain information about them, however, is to grow their cells in the laboratory. Cells that are grown in laboratory culture dishes are referred to as *in vitro* cells, from the Latin expression meaning "in glass." ("In plastic" would be more accurate these days, but both etymology and Alice favor glass, and so shall we.) Whatever they are grown in, in vitro cultures are cells that were removed from an organism. Cells that are still in the organism are referred to as *in vivo*, meaning "in life"—although that is misleading, since the in vitro cells are also alive, if the researcher is careful. The degree of care required in each case distinguishes in vitro from in vivo in a deeper sense than you might think. The organism is the natural environment for its cells, and, in general, they survive longer and with far less planning and attention from the researcher when they are left in vivo. Cells in vitro are never exactly the same as those in the organism. Growing our tiger lily cells in the laboratory, however, simplifies our job: We know exactly what we did and exactly what the conditions were when we did it.

In vitro and in vivo experiments have different implications as well. Results from in vitro experiments aren't necessarily applicable to in vivo treatments, because cells grow differently in culture.

Even if their behavior in vitro exactly mimicked that in vivo, treatments that work in the culture dish would not necessarily be effective in vivo. A drug that effectively treats cancer cells in a culture dish could be toxic to other types of cells in the body. The drug could kill the cancer, but kill the rest of the body, too.

In most experiments in vitro, the results serve mainly as a screening for clinical possibilities. But, fortunately for us, when we look specifically at aging, the in vitro information (for example, the Hayflick limit) correlates well with the in vivo information (for example, the life span of the species the cells were taken from).[1] Any technique that alters aging in culture or any understanding of aging based on cultured cells is very likely to have a direct bearing on aging of the organism in vivo.

Laboratory studies of cells in vitro support the theory that telomeric mechanism causes aging: Cells age because the telomere shortens. Telomere shortening is related to the number of cell generations and accurately predicts when the cells will age. The greater the number of cell generations that have occurred, the shorter the telomeres; the shorter the telomeres, the older the behavior of the cell. In the final stages of telomere shortening, the cell changes its pattern of gene expression, slows its rate of division, then stops dividing at all, and then finally dies.

The length of telomeres decreases directly with the number of generations. On the average, cells lose fifty base pairs, or about eight TTAGGGs, per division. That loss is not the result of random DNA attrition (occurring just anywhere in the chromosome); nor is it simply rearrangement of DNA from the telomere to nontelomeric sites (so that the telomeric sequences moved elsewhere in the chromosome). The loss is of TTAGGGs from the telomere.

How good is the telomere as a predictor of cellular aging? It is the best predictor we know. Put whimsically—but accurately—it is a better predictor of aging than is your age itself. To explore this peculiar irony, we need to understand the relationship between aging and age. When we take fibroblasts from a person's skin and grow them in culture, we know that person's age. We might expect that fibroblasts from a newborn child will live longer in culture than those from a one-hundred-year-old person, and that is exactly what happens: We have greater success trying to grow cells from a child than from a centenarian. When we measure cellular aging—biochemical function and ability to divide and grow—cells drawn from older donors don't do as well as those from younger donors.

Although there is usually an excellent correlation between a person's age and how old their cells act, that is not always the case.

Each of us has occasionally met individuals who looked far younger,

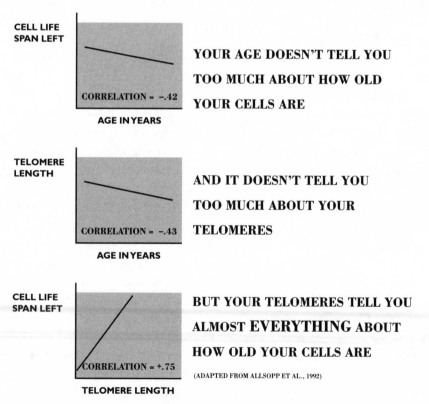

CELL LIFE SPAN LEFT

CORRELATION = −.42

AGE IN YEARS

YOUR AGE DOESN'T TELL YOU TOO MUCH ABOUT HOW OLD YOUR CELLS ARE

TELOMERE LENGTH

CORRELATION = −.43

AGE IN YEARS

AND IT DOESN'T TELL YOU TOO MUCH ABOUT YOUR TELOMERES

CELL LIFE SPAN LEFT

CORRELATION = +.75

TELOMERE LENGTH

BUT YOUR TELOMERES TELL YOU ALMOST EVERYTHING ABOUT HOW OLD YOUR CELLS ARE

(ADAPTED FROM ALLSOPP ET AL., 1992)

Fig. 4.1

or older, than their years. Not only is there variation in aging as we assess it—intuitively and at a glance—but the same is true of any measure of aging that we pick. People vary in the rate at which they age; should we be surprised that the same is true of their cells? Just as being sixty years old doesn't mean that you look exactly the same age as all other sixty-year-olds, so too, having sixty-year-old skin doesn't mean that your cells have exactly the same number of generations left as every other sixty-year-old skin cell. To the contrary, fibroblasts drawn from several people of identical chronological age will vary not only in how old they act initially, but in how they will continue to age in the culture dish. If the number of years lived is not the best predictor of aging, what is?

The best predictor of subsequent aging is the telomere length.[2] Fibroblasts with short telomeres, even if they are drawn from a young donor, will soon show cell aging. Those fibroblasts with longer telomeres, even if they are drawn from an old donor, will take longer to show cell aging. Aging is not a process that occurs passively as a result of living a certain number of years, but is a process that occurs as telomeric shortening allows entropy to take you apart. That process may take years, but it is absolutely dependent upon telomeric shortening and the defenses that it controls. The best correlation is therefore between telomere length and aging, not between chronological age and aging. You are only as old as your telomeres.

ELEPHANTS AND MICE

It was six men of Indostan, To learning much inclined,
Who went to see the Elephant (Though all of them were blind),
That each by observation might satisfy his mind.

JOHN SAXE, "THE BLIND MEN AND THE ELEPHANT"

When we consider aging, whether we look at different species or at different aspects of the aging process, we should remember that finally, it is still one common process throughout. Aging is like the elephant in the parable about the blind men. Running his hands over the elephant's trunklike legs, one thought it was a tree; feeling the trunk, another thought it a snake; finding its broad sides, still another believed it to be a wall. Yet it remained a single, solid elephant. Researchers of aging have focused on DNA damage, free radicals, mitochondria, and other aspects of aging; they have studied flies, fish, mice, and humans; and although they have reached different conclusions about the nature of aging, it is still one process.

Even though every living thing differs in how and when it ages, those differences are not profound ones. Some are merely quantitative: Some animals age in a day, some in a century, but they all age. All backboned animals (vertebrates)—such as ourselves, other mammals, birds, reptiles, amphibians, and fish—share most of the same metabolic machinery and have identical telomere sequences.

Organisms more distant from us in form and evolution, such as yeast, bacteria, and viruses, may age differently or even not at all, but they still teach us something about our own aging. Although we have only sampled a few dozen species—a few parts of the elephant—we have finally realized that we are not dealing with different mechanisms of aging for each species: The mechanisms are the same, even though the shapes may be different. There is a single, almost universal aging process. There is only one elephant.

All living creatures face the same problem of replicating their chromosomes without losing pieces of themselves every time. With each replication, a small piece of the end of the chromosome is lost, leaving one of the two daughter cells without part of a telomere. Progressively shorter with each generation, the chromosome threatens to disappear altogether. Then how can life continue? How can we have inherited chromosomes from our parents at all, let alone from an ancestry stretching back three billion years?

Nature has invented at least three solutions to the problem. The first is to avoid the problem altogether by not having chromosome ends. After all, why have ends to begin with if it is so much trouble to copy them? Why not form a chromosome that has no end? That is exactly what many bacteria and viruses do—form circular chromosomes. Their chromosomes are rings without ends, so they don't lose pieces during replication. The common bacteria found in your intestine, *E coli*, does just that, as does the virus mentioned already, SV40.

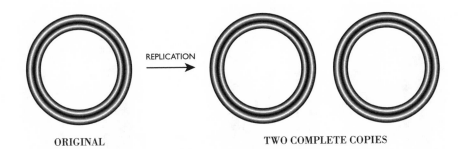

ORIGINAL   TWO COMPLETE COPIES

**The first solution:
a ring chromosome**

Fig. 4.2

In both cases, the chromosomes are small circles, without telomeres at all. When they are copied, the DNA polymerases—Xerox machines of the genetic realm and responsible for replicating the entire chromosome—simply move around the entire ring until they finally return to the place where they began. There is no loss of DNA, no telomere shortening, and no aging. These organisms—bacteria, viruses, and others—are immortal in the sense that they do not age. They can die by the billions, but they do not succumb to an internal clock that shuts them down as the chromosome shortens. The chromosomes remain ageless rings, without a telomere.

A second solution is to have a special protein at the end of the chromosome that determines the starting point for copying the DNA and doesn't allow any shortening. Replication begins at the special starter protein and progresses without any loss of telomere; the end of the chromosome is copied faithfully every time. This mechanism is typical of some viruses such as the adenoviruses that cause sore throat, bronchitis, and pneumonia. Their chromosomes have ends, but they never shorten; they remain immortal. Your immune system recognizes them and kills them reliably, and yet these viruses return with the seasons, and perhaps will forever.

The third solution—and the one that your germ cells use—is probably universal among organisms with nuclei. There is no ring or special protein lock on the end of the telomere, but rather, the telomere is allowed to shorten and the lost pieces are then replaced. In this case the telomere that caps the end of the chromosome is purposely without

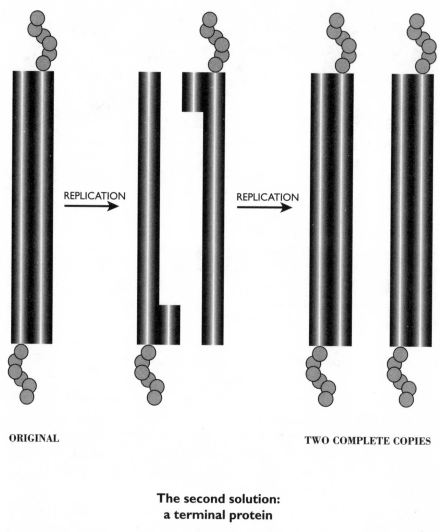

ORIGINAL   TWO COMPLETE COPIES

**The second solution:
a terminal protein**

Fig. 4.3

any actual genes; the loss can be replaced predictably and uniformly by using a telomerase "stamp" that re-creates exactly what was lost. The stamp adds a series of predictable and identical sequences, restoring the lost bases and restoring telomere length.

For many organisms, especially those that are one-celled and immortal, this mechanism operates faithfully, and it is found in every cell of every organism of the species that use it. Yeasts,[3] for instance, are usually immortal. They divide repeatedly and have done so since early

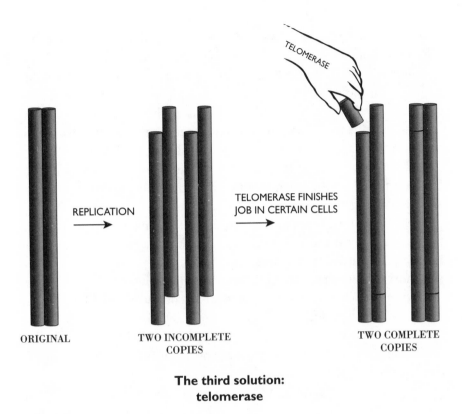

**The third solution:
telomerase**

Fig. 4.4

in the history of life on our planet. They express telomerase and reextend their telomeres using the third solution described above.

At least normal yeasts do. There is a mutated form, est 1 (for "ever shortening telomere"), that gradually loses telomeric DNA, senesces, and dies.[4] Once again, the rule holds: Telomere loss triggers aging. Even in yeasts that have survived since life began, immortal and ageless, once we allow the telomere to shorten, they rapidly succumb, as they never had for more than three billion years, to aging.[5] The yeast dies of old age and—relative to its previous immortality—it does so within the blink of an eye.

All because the telomere shortened.

Tetrahymena, a relative of the paramecium, must replace its lost telomere sequences (in this case TTGGGG, rather than your own TTAGGG sequence) continuously in order to stay alive. If, however, the telomerase in tetrahymena becomes inactive, the organism ages and dies.[6]

Normally, whether in yeasts, tetrahymena, or human germ cells, the telomere shortens with each replication, the chromosomes lose bases, telomerase adds them back onto the telomere, and the organism remains in business. The operation is a careful balance: If there are too many bases, the organism will have wasted its resources producing endless, needless telomere bases; but if there are too few bases, the organism dies as the telomere runs out and genes are lost.

This balance foreshadows a more interesting one that occurs in your own mortal cells—the balance between getting cancer on the one hand and early aging on the other.

In one-celled organisms, however, the balance may be more elementary. An immortal cell is between the "rock" of a telomere that is too long (wasting cellular resources) and the "hard place" of one that is too short (and the risk of death from cellular aging). It can guarantee "immortality" by spending its metabolic energy on building a long telomere but then still lose its life needlessly to a competitor that is "leaner and meaner," or it can have a short, efficient telomere, but risk using up its telomeric safety net and dying needlessly, perhaps in the midst of plenty.

It is a careful, uncertain, and continuous balance that the cell must maintain: just so long a telomere, just so much telomerase. From moment to moment, the organism is adjusting to the feedback of metabolic danger signals, DNA damage, and available resources, which they must attend too in order to pass on their genes and survive.

Or perhaps long telomeres aren't merely wasteful; maybe they pose some other disadvantage to one-celled organisms. After all, how much harder can it be to maintain a long telomere than a short one? The same number of bases need to be added with each (telomere-shortening) division. Is there some more important need that a relatively short telomere serves for one-celled organisms? Long, unwieldy telomeres might make it more difficult to duplicate the chromosome or to manipulate the chromosome to express some of the genes. Or perhaps short telomeres help prevent cells with DNA damage from dividing. As we will see, this would be similar to the purpose it serves for larger, multicelled organisms, like human beings. No one yet knows the answers to these questions. Whatever the advantage, metabolic savings, ease of duplication, gene expression, or safety net in the face of DNA damage, telomeres are not kept needlessly long.

Organisms with more than one cell experience the same problem of shortening telomeres as single cells; but multicellular organisms also have another problem: cancer. They address the threat of shortening telomeres in roughly the same way that unicellular organisms do but with a twist: The telomere bases are replaced, *but only in germ cells*. (If somatic cells relengthened their telomeres, they would be able to ignore the needs of their neighbors and grow unchecked at the expense of the rest of the body. In one-celled organisms, cells that grow unchecked are merely competitive; but when cells in a multicellular organism grow unchecked, they are cancer cells.)

By itself, cell growth is not destructive—in fact, it is crucial to the multicellular organism. Not only must groups of cells multiply to form organs, but some must be replaced continuously for you to survive. Bones are formed and re-formed by carefully balanced regulation of bone-forming cells and bone-destroying cells; miles of blood vessels are formed; neurons form connections across remarkable distances—as much as fifty thousand times their cell body lengths—and do so precisely. Skin cells are constantly replaced, as are red blood cells, white blood cells, cells of the intestinal lining, and others damaged in trauma or infection.

All of these cells must act in exact coordination with the other cells that make up the body. Each cell has a set of blueprints—the chromosomes—and a subset of genes whose expression must respond not only to its own needs but to those of the rest of the body. Hormones, nutrients, electrical signals, local messengers, all play roles in determining what each cell does and whether or not it should divide. Each of your cells responds to orders and does so specifically and obediently if you are to survive and compete.

A cell that does not respond correctly to these "social cues" becomes transformed from a normal cell to a potentially dangerous cell, a transformation that occurs when the regulatory mechanisms controlling gene expression are damaged by viruses, radiation, or carcinogens. These cells that no longer support their normal neighbors may multiply without check or restraint. They harm other cells by taking away the body's resources—and giving nothing useful in return—by invading other organs, and by preventing normal function. These are cancer cells in the making.

How does your body prevent cancer? Normally, your cells respond to the social messages of other cells and of the body in general. But what happens if a cell no longer responds? To begin with, it has the same resources that we have already encountered in other contexts. Its first defense is a brake on cell division: The cell will refuse to divide when it finds DNA damage; a special "braking" protein, p53, stops DNA replication and stimulates repair. But what if there is a failure in this brake? Each cell has a deadman switch, a genetic time bomb, that kills the cell if it continues to divide.[7] That time bomb is the telomere, which works in two ways: by shutting down the cell whenever it detects DNA damage, and by limiting overall replication (with or without damage). The telomere triggers the same "damage" signal when it shortens as the cell divides too many times (as cancer cells do). The telomere clock counts down with each replication and shuts down the cells.

The DDBPs that normally bind to damaged DNA also bind to the telomere when it shortens to a certain point and shut down replication. When there is either gross damage to the DNA or more subtle damage in the form of a cell's inability to respond correctly to other cells, these proteins block DNA synthesis and cell division. In both cases, the cell cycle brakes to a halt and cancer cells are shut down and prevented from growing. That usually works, but not always. If the cancer cell continues to divide after the telomere is gone, wholesale genetic destruction and, finally, cell death ensue. But if the cell manages to reset the telomere—to turn off the time bomb and continue dividing without losing its telomeres—it becomes malignant.

The cell monitors itself for DNA damage and telomere length. The brakes will be applied unless its DNA is intact and it has a long enough telomere. Cancer cells not only have damaged DNA[8] but evade the checkpoint "brake" *and* relengthen their telomeres by expressing telomerase. These two events—checkpoint evasion and telomerase expression—are the two hurdles that cancer cells must overcome.[9] In other words, they must ignore the brake on division that normally responds to DNA damage and they must avoid continued shortening of their telomere in order to become immortal.

Random damage is not enough to cause cancer. The cell can overcome the first hurdle only if there is *specific* damage to the brake—the checkpoint—that controls cell division. Cancers result from damage, or an inherited error, somewhere in this braking mechanism, whether to p53—as do 70 percent of colon cancers, 50 percent of lung cancers, and 40 percent of breast cancers—or to one of the related proteins that together act to stop unbridled cell division.

The second hurdle, telomere shortening, is more difficult for cancer cells to pass. Only 1 in perhaps 3 million cells do so and survive. Cancer cells have to do more than just ignore the loss of telomere repeats and the signals that order the cell to stop dividing. If it does evade the checkpoint, the telomere continues to lose bases. Soon the subtelomere is lost, followed by loss of functional genes; then the cell stops functioning and finally dies. To remain viable, the cancer cell must not only evade the checkpoint, but also turn on telomerase and reconstruct at least some of the telomere that caps the end of its chromosome.

Why are cancer cells so dangerous? Multicellular organisms cannot tolerate these "sociopathic" entities that roam unimpeded and that do not know their place in the society of cells. The importance for the organism is obvious; it requires enough years to reproduce and raise offspring. But beyond that, evolution loses interest. The telomeric clock in cells must be short enough to preclude an outbreak of cancer in the young, but long enough to allow the organism to live to reproduce. Evolution has struck a balance, giving you just enough time to reproduce and ensure a likely success for your offspring. After that, you begin to age and die.

But the same mechanism that lowers the chances of cancer also has the side effect of causing aging. Aging is the side effect of preventing irresponsible cell growth. Cal Harley puts it succinctly: "Cellular senescence confers a strict level of growth control and reduces the probability of cancer."[10] Aging is not something that just happens as you get older: It is designed to occur so that cancer rarely does.

But not all multicellular organisms use the exact same clock mechanism. For instance, in the fly *Drosophila*, the cells do not divide after adulthood; the fly has no replacement parts: There are no stem cells, no generic cells from which to produce other cells lost to infection or trauma, and its telomeres are markedly different. In effect, the fly's cells are already senescent, and it has no problem with cancer.[11]

How do telomeres differ among vertebrates? No one yet knows. But we have good reason to believe that the clock mechanism works similarly among all vertebrates, because the telomere sequence is invariant and they share a common tendency toward cancer. However, there are inevitably differences, for several reasons.

Cell replacement occurs in most species, but the methods vary. Some species, such as the housefly, have no replacement at all. In others, when it occurs, cell replacement takes two forms: replacement of special cell lines—such as your red blood cells and your colon cells—or regeneration of whole body parts. The human body continuously replaces colon cells and blood cells; the risk of cancer in these dividing cells is high. Neurons, at the other extreme, do not divide in the adult organism and therefore present a low risk of cancer. Regeneration of body parts in humans is remarkable not only because it is so rare—it occurs far less with us than it does with amphibians and reptiles—but also because of what the cells must do. Cells responsible for regeneration must be capable of setting aside their day-to-day responsibilities and drastically altering their gene expression. To regenerate a limb, for example, requires more than just producing a single category of cells, such as blood or colon cells; bone, muscle, tendon, skin, and other parts of the body also have to be produced.

Both cell line replacement and regeneration bring on the additional risk that these cells may escape their limits and become cancerous. Different species vary in their potential for cell transformation, and so are likely to vary in their mechanisms of preventing cell transformation, the emphasis and strength of the braking mechanisms, and in how the cell "reads" its telomeres.

Another source of cancer that varies among different species is DNA damage done by free radicals and other biochemical sources. Some vertebrates—those with higher metabolic rates, for example—produce more free radicals than others; some ingest more toxins that cross-link or otherwise damage their DNA; and some are more exposed to high-energy photons. Viral infection also varies profoundly among species. X rays injure any DNA, but viruses are picky. The virus that causes cervical cancer in humans is innocuous in the frog, and the virus that causes leukemia in the cat doesn't bother the monkey.

Because it has the same purpose, we expect the telomere mechanism to work the same way in other animals that it does in us. There should be a correlation—with some allowances for slightly different cellular mechanisms in different species—between life span and telomere length. Unfortunately, we know next to nothing about the telomere length in most species.

Even in mice—a laboratory animal that we know a great deal

about—we don't yet know the telomere length. Mice have a shorter life span, so their telomeres might be expected to be shorter than ours. On the other hand, their metabolic rate is higher, so their cell turnover—and hence telomere shortening rate—is higher than ours. But the only thing we know so far is that the terminal restriction fragment (TRF), rather than the telomere, is longer than that in humans,[12] even though mice have shorter life spans.[13]

While we suspect that telomere length determines the maximum life span in different species, we are not yet certain of it.[14] It may be that the variance of the telomere will be more important than the average length—as was discussed above (see Figure 3.8). Or perhaps the rate of shortening—how many base pairs are lost per division—will be far more significant than length of the telomere at birth or conception. Likewise, if cells turn over more quickly, the aging rate will also be rapid, even if telomeres are relatively long. It is equally possible that in some animals the engines of aging—free radicals, for instance—will be so powerful, and will act so rapidly, that aging will occur early despite relatively long telomeres. No one yet knows if that is so, nor do we know what implications these effects would have for human aging and its reversal. What is known is how well telomere length correlates with aging in human beings and how well the telomeres explain aging, cancer, and cell immortality.

A PIECE OF WORK

What a piece of work is man!

—HAMLET, II.ii

INTRODUCTION

Some cells age more quickly than others. Not every cell ages directly, but all cells are affected by the overall aging of the organism. Some cells lose their blood supplies; others drown in waste products that are no longer filtered or broken down by distant cells; still others are injured by trauma and infection as their neighbors lose the ability to defend them from such damage. Some cells, such as those of progerics, are born already old; others age directly as their telomeres shorten, or indirectly as cells around them age and fail. To paraphrase Shakespeare, in the context of cell aging: "Some cells are born aged, some achieve age, some have aging thrust upon them."

In this section, we will examine normal human tissues and how the telomere *directly* causes aging in them, as well as an important exception, the sperm cell, whose telomeres do not shorten and which does not age at all. We will also consider several diseases that have a direct bearing on aging and the telomere—among them cancer and the two major progeric syndromes (Werner's and Hutchinson-Gilford). The choice of cancer might be obvious (in light of the discussion in the last section and the vital relation of cancer to aging) but the relevance to aging of other diseases will be less obvious. For instance, what does Down's syndrome, the most common form of mental retardation, have to do with aging? What can the AIDS virus, which causes the veritable destruction of the immune system, reveal to us about aging? And can an understanding of aging help us understand, treat, or even cure AIDS? We have answers to only some of these questions, but examining diseases in which the supply of certain cells is depleted will shed light on the aging process in general.

First, in order to explore the aging changes of somatic cells, we will look at sperm cells, which are germ cells and do not age.

NORMAL HUMAN TISSUE

Sperm Cells

Sperm are more easily studied than eggs because they are more plentiful and accessible than their female counterparts. Consequently, much more is known about sperm than about eggs. Sperm cells have longer telomeres than somatic cells[15] and they do not shorten with age;[16] the length of a telomere in germ cells from a newborn child is the same as that from a one-hundred-year-old man. Neither years nor the body's aging affects these cells nor their telomeres, even though they are carried in the same environment, bathed in the same blood, and subject to the same aging influences as somatic cells. How can these cells, which have the same genes, the same number of years of life, the same free radicals, the same trauma and infections, the same exposure to almost everything as the body's other cells, not age? Sperm cells continue to divide throughout the male life span without any indication of either telomere shortening or aging.

The lack of aging in sperm cells provides two important conclusions for us: first, that aging is a result of telomerase expression, which we have already seen; and second, that aging is equally a result of gene expression, which has a far-reaching implication. The second conclusion implies that sperm cells don't age because even though they have the *same genes* as somatic cells, the sperm cells *express the genes differently*.

Aging—and survival itself—is not just a matter of which genes you have, but also of how they are expressed. We age differently from tortoises, because we have different genes. But human somatic cells and germ cells have the same genes and yet they *still* age differently. Our maximum age span is not limited solely by our having the right genes to defend against free radicals, but by how—and for how long—those genes express themselves. The fact that germ cells never age isn't very important. What is important is that they never age even though *they have the same genes as the rest of your cells*. The "cause" of aging, then, is a particular pattern of gene expression—senescent gene expression—and the trigger for senescent gene expression is telomere shortening. Sperm cells don't age because they reliably express telomerase and therefore continue their normal pattern of gene expression.[17] Thus, human genes are already up to the task of indefinitely defending our cells against aging. We don't need some special gene, whether found in tortoises or created in the laboratory, to prevent aging; we need to modify the expression of those genes—which the telomere does in our germ cells.

Sperm cells tell us that the genes we already possess, properly expressed, can maintain our cells without aging.

Fibroblasts

The body is primarily made up of somatic cells that do not express telomerase and that age normally. Historically, the first and most studied example of this is the fibroblast; it is the classic example of a cell in which primary aging changes occur. This cell, deep in your skin, divides whenever necessary, replacing the framework that holds you together, forming a solid layer of protection and support around your body. And as this cell ages, it demonstrates predictable changes in function, the most reliable being a decreasing ability to divide.[18] Whether grown in culture, or allowed to live, grow, and divide in the body, fibroblasts lose about twenty telomere bases per year,[19] and their gene expression changes as they come to the end of the telomere.

Our interest is not in chronological age, but in the aging process itself: in how healthy we are. The correlation between age in years and fibroblast aging is not exact, the correlation between age in years and telomere length is also not exact, but the correlation between telomere length and fibroblast aging is almost perfect.[20] But even if the telomere is the best *measure* of cell aging, *what determines how long it is?* The most important factor is the number of times the cell divides, but what makes cells divide in the first place?

How old your cells are isn't determined by age in years, but—again paraphrasing George Burns—by the mileage. The mileage, for a fibroblast, includes sun exposure, trauma, infections, and anything else that increases the "odometer" setting—the number of divisions. The mileage is also influenced by your genes: Some of us have better pigment protection from ultraviolet rays, better reflexes, or a stronger immune system. And even with the same number of divisions, some fibroblasts might lose more base pairs in each division than others do. However, your age in years is related to how old your fibroblasts are because it gives you more time to be exposed to damage. Your lifestyle—no matter what your chronological age—is also related to the aging of your cells, because the more they have been damaged, the more they have needed to divide to replace the losses. That's why your skin reflects different degrees of aging, depending on where you look: The skin exposed to the sun and wind—on your neck, for example—looks older than skin elsewhere. The fibroblasts don't age because you are sixty, or because you went sunbathing, or because you are fairskinned. They age because they were damaged, they divided, the clock ran down, and their gene expression altered.

Thus, the years, the damage, and the cell divisions all play a role in cell aging, but the telomere is the final common denominator, the universal yardstick, for fibroblasts and other skin cells.

Red Blood Cells

Blood comprises fluid—water, proteins, salts, etc.—and two major types of cells—red and white. Normal, healthy blood has about five hundred red cells for every white one. Red cells live an average of four months and are constantly replaced from stem cells in your bone marrow, which divide as necessary. "As necessary" covers innumerable situations. The replenishment of red cells by the stem cells in your bone marrow involves a delicate, wavering balance, subject to the effects of blood loss (menstrual and traumatic), removal of old blood cells (usually by the spleen), availability of crucial nutrients (for instance, iron, folate, and cyanocobalamin), blood flow through the kidneys (which make hormones that regulate production of red cells), availability of oxygen to the body's tissues (for instance, changes that occur when you move to high altitudes), genetic abnormalities (for instance, sickle-cell disease), pregnancy, and other factors. The output of red blood cells can vary as much as sixfold (that is, the maximum production can increase to six times the minimum) even in the healthy person, depending on these factors.[21]

The process is not simple, although the outline is. There are, on the one hand, forces that urge the stem cell to divide more often (and increase the number of red cells in the blood); on the other hand, there are forces that put the brake on stem cell division. The balance between these two competing inputs results in the day-to-day red blood cell concentration (the hematocrit). However, there might be another factor involved—telomere length.

The cells in your marrow that make red blood cells must have divided numerous times to produce all the red cells that you need in a lifetime. The best current estimate is that between 1,000 and 3,500 cell divisions have occurred to make each of the blood cells of a sixty-year-old, compared with only 20 to 50 cell divisions that had occurred by the time of birth.[22] But fibroblasts can only divide about 50 times after birth. Do the stem cells that produce the red cells avoid the Hayflick limit by expressing telomerase after birth or do they simply have an astoundingly high Hayflick limit? If they express telomerase, we might expect telomere lengths to stay the same over the years, but they don't. They shorten like those of other cells, losing about thirty-three base pairs per year.[23]

What if that loss was the result of a balance in which at least small amounts of telomerase were expressed and, although the telomere shortened, it did so more slowly because of the telomerase partly making up for the loss? Researchers have looked into that possibility, but no one has yet found even a trace of telomerase activity in the red blood stem cells, despite their stunning turnover.[24]

Though the estimates of the number of cell divisions could be wrong, if they are correct, then blood stem cells would have to have a much higher Hayflick limit than fibroblasts do. If that is so, then either the stem cell telomere must be longer than that of fibroblasts—but stem cells appear to lack the telomerase they would need to make it longer!—or the stem cells must lose fewer base pairs per cell division than do fibroblasts—but they both have the same problem in duplicating the end of the chromosome that all human cells have and should lose base pairs at the same rate! Perhaps telomerase *is* expressed, but only until birth; we might be born with a huge number of stem cells, which divided thousands of times because they had telomerase prenatally, each with a completely wound clock, capable of producing red blood cells for a lifetime.

But no matter when your stem cells expressed telomerase, it would be an enormous risk. If they expressed too little telomerase, you might not have the stem cells you need to produce red blood cells for a lifetime. If they expressed too much telomerase, then your risk of cancer would go up, as precancerous cells were given license to divide more. If they expressed too little, you would be anemic; too much, you would have leukemia. Once again, as we did in the last chapter when we discussed how aging and cancer are related, we see the dangerously narrow path that all multicellular organisms must take between a rock and a hard place: too few old cells on the one hand, too many cancerous ones on the other.

White Cells

About one in every five hundred blood cells is a white cell, though the actual number of white cells is far higher than this suggests. Most of these leukocytes are not in the blood at all, but rather in the tissue, outside of the blood vessels; those that we see in the blood are on their way to other locations. Leukocytes are a motley collection of various cells, all vaguely immune in function. They are responsible for attacking intruders, recognizing foreign material and damaged cells, and cleaning up inflammation. They are the soldiers and the housekeeping cells of the body.

White cells frequently die doing their jobs, although some may live for as long as the body does. Like red cells, white cells are replaced from the stem cells of the bone marrow. And their telomeres usually shorten with age.[25] The rate of loss (about forty base pairs per year) is comparable with that of other cells. This forms an interesting backdrop for diseases, such as Down's syndrome or AIDS, in which white blood cells age faster than they do in normal individuals. The astounding turnover of white blood cells in AIDS, more than a billion cells a day,[26] results in shortened telomeres and rapid aging—and exhaustion—of the stem cells that try to replace this loss. As we will see below, this has intriguing therapeutic potential.

Do white blood cells express telomerase? Most don't, but a recent report from researchers at McMaster University in Canada and the Geron Corporation in California confirms that certain very rare young white blood cells do just that.[27] Trace amounts of telomerase have been found, not in the earliest stem cells, but in a restricted subset of white cells in the bone marrow and even in circulating blood.

Despite this rare exception, as the telomere shortens in normal white blood cells, it signals the cell to slow further division and replacement of cells, and it no longer protects the end of the chromosome from destruction and from "sticking" to other chromosomes. As a result, there is an increase in chromosomal abnormalities with age.[28]

Blood Vessels

The cells that line the walls of your vascular system, your blood vessels, are subject to constant stress. The stresses are small, but repeated continuously with every heartbeat. Just as large wires can finally be broken by repeated folding, so can these small, repeated stresses damage your blood vessels. Your ribs and the bones of your feet are commonly subject to stress fractures in which similar small, repeated stresses (for instance, a day of severe coughing or unaccustomed walking) serve to break them. Throughout your life, the blood vessels are subject to these stresses. As your heart beats, sending waves of pressure down the blood vessels, the walls are repeatedly stretched and pulled an average of once a second for your entire life. Cells that are lost as a result of this stress must be replaced without interrupting the vessel wall. An error causes a weakening of the wall, which results either in a tear—with bleeding into the wall—or a ballooning aneurysm. The aneurysm, whatever the type, results all too frequently in death. When these cells succumb to stress, they must be replaced reliably because the organism cannot afford an error.

The stress on these cells determines how often they die, which determines how often they need to be replaced. Each time a cell has to divide and replace its neighbor, its telomere shortens. For example, the cells from the veins undergo far less stress than those from arteries, and need less replacement of damaged cells. The arteries have the continual, pulsatile stress of blood pressure rising and falling with each beat of your heart. Therefore, even though both kinds of cells begin with the same size telomeres, the cells that line adult veins have longer telomeres than those from adult arteries.[29] Although the mechanisms of disease are complex, this seemingly simple observation helps explain why vascular disease accompanies aging: cells with greater demands for replacement have a higher rate of turnover, shorter telomeres, and faster cell aging.

Other Cells

The same process occurs in almost every cell line. Kidney cells show aging as their telomeres shorten;[30] so do mucosal cells from the colon.[31] But loss does not occur in a few white blood cells, or in cancer cells.

When grown in cultures, normal cells can be "transformed" into cancer cells—by genetic damage or viral infection—and they neither age nor shorten their telomeres. Perhaps the best known of these is the tumor-derived HeLa line (named for Henrietta Lacks, who donated the original cervical cancer cells forty years ago). This line of immortal cancer cells can be grown indefinitely, with no indication of cellular aging.[32] While normal human fibroblast cultures must be restarted periodically from a fresh biopsy, as they age and die in the laboratory, HeLa cells can be—and are—passed from lab to lab and grown for decades, with no indication of a limit to the number of times that they can divide. They are cancer cells and they are immortal.

The same expression of telomerase seen in HeLa cells is seen in virally "transformed" cells (transformed into tumor cells by a virus such as *SV40* or *Ad5*) if they become immortal.[33] *SV40* viral infection is sufficient to extend the life span of the cells slightly, but they still age and die unless they can express telomerase, which renders them immortal. The ability to reextend the telomere is the passport to immortalization of virally infected cells.

HUMAN CELLS IN DISEASE

Vascular Disease

Atherosclerosis is the primary cause of cardiovascular disease in developed countries.[34] Although contributing factors are legion, the process begins with an injury that is due to either repeated hemodynamic stress[35] (discussed above), infection, genetic disorders, or trauma. The injured area responds by increasing cell turnover as it attempts to replace lost and damaged cells. Those areas are especially prone to cell aging because all this turnover has caused the cells to lose telomere length faster than normal cells do.

Hypertension, the most serious and ongoing stress for arterial vessel cells—like other sources of vessel injury—causes the cells of the vessel walls to divide at an abnormally high rate, which results in premature telomere shortening and early aging for these cells.[36] In most common cases, wall injury results in not only increased cell turnover, but also increased inflammation and accumulation of cholesterol plaques.[37] This narrows the vessel and finally brings about the death of tissues that depend on the blood flow. Arteries of the heart, for instance, become narrowed with plaque and are finally too small to support the demands of the heart muscle, which then dies. If crucial areas or a sufficient amount of cardiac muscle dies, then so does the patient.

Plaques and vessel narrowing are not the only pathology of vessels. Most aneurysms are also caused by atherosclerosis.[38] The cells that line these diseased arteries are frequently damaged and have a high rate of turnover.[39]

In comparing cells from healthy vessel walls with cells from areas with plaque, it is clear that cells from areas with low stress and that are not prone to plaques—such as the internal thoracic artery—have longer telomeres than cells from areas that have high hemodynamic stress and are prone to plaques—such as the iliac artery. When we attempt to grow these cells in culture, the cells coming from damaged areas die out sooner, and the nearer the cells are to areas of plaque and stress, the less capable they are of normal growth.[40] Cells from atherosclerotic areas have telomere lengths typical of aging cells rather than being normal for the age of the individual.[41] If you are only forty, but have a strong genetic predilection for heart disease, then parts of your arteries are already twice that old.

This conclusion is also supported by the fact that patients who begin life with short telomeres (progerics) have a high incidence of arterial disease, which develops before age ten, not because of decades of high cholesterol or hemodynamic stress, but rather because of their shortened telomeres. Generically, these patients—with artherosclerosis or progeria—are examples of a group of diseases caused by inappropriately short telomeres. Some diseases in this group—the two major progeric syndromes—are almost exclusively a result of this defect. With others, like Down's syndrome and AIDS, only a part of their pathology is explained by the shortened telomeres.

DISEASES ASSOCIATED WITH SHORT TELOMERES

Hutchinson-Gilford Syndrome
Hutchinson-Gilford syndrome is a disease caused by short telomeres. These children—they never live to be adults—have remarkable pathology, which mostly parallels normal aging, but in an extremely and tragically accelerated fashion.[42] The parallels are not exact, but are still overwhelming, so that the disease has the appearance of a normal aging process gone wild. The cells from children with this syndrome are less able to replicate[43] and their telomeres are shorter[44] than those of normal children. Their parents, however, have normal telomere lengths for their age. Most likely, the telomeres of the father's sperm had, due to mutation, undergone inappropriate shortening prior to fertilization and his child inherited a short telomere at conception.[45] The telomeres don't shorten at a faster rate—they are just shorter to begin with.

Compared with those of normal children, the telomeres of Hutchinson-Gilford children at birth are like those of a ninety-year-old. This is a rough estimate, obtained by subtracting the subtelomere length from the total terminal restriction fragment (TRF) length and comparing it with the telomere lengths of normal people at various ages. Few of

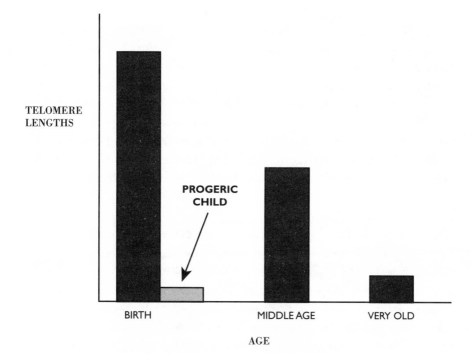

PROGERICS HAVE OLD CELLS AT BIRTH
(ADAPTED FROM ALLSOPP ET AL., 1992)

Fig. 4.5

these children have had their TRFs measured, and none have yet had just the TTAGGG repeats measured.[46] However, while a specific cellular age for Hutchinson-Gilford children may be inexact, clearly their bodies are remarkably old before they have ever had a chance to be young.

Werner's Syndrome

We would expect that Werner's syndrome, in which aging begins in early adulthood, should also be—by analogy to Hutchinson-Gilford syndrome—a disease caused by moderately shortened telomeres. Their cells certainly show earlier Hayflick limits compared with cells from people who age normally,[47] but contrary to our expectation, their telomeres are not shorter to begin with (at least not in some patients). What likely happens is that their telomeres shorten faster than do normal telomeres. Their telomeric clocks begin with the same time as a normal clock, but they run faster.

The story is, of course, not as simple as this. Werner's syndrome cells are abnormal in other ways. Their cell cycle is slower; their mutation rates are higher by as much as ten to one hundred times; and they don't show the usual pattern of enzyme changes that normal aging cells do.[48]

Progeria often refers only to Hutchinson-Gilford syndrome, excluding Werner's syndrome. This distinction may be appropriate, for though Werner's patients appear old, the mechanism that causes this disease is not necessarily the alteration of the telomeric clock that occurs with the children with Hutchinson-Gilford syndrome.

Down's Syndrome

A person with Down's syndrome has an extra copy of chromosome 21—hence the disease's other name, trisomy 21—and is retarded mentally. However, the typical Down's syndrome child has other problems. Among them are frequent infections that occur because the telomeres of their immune cells—for example, their white blood cells—shorten faster than do normal immune cells.[49] The white blood cells of these patients have shorter telomeres and the patients often succumb to infections as though their immune systems were old. However, Down's syndrome is not the disease that exhibits the worst immune dysfunction. Instead, that is found in disorders involving certain genetic deletions and with some viral infections, the worst of which is HIV.

AIDS

In HIV, a virus invades a cell, rewrites part of the genetic library, and forces the cell to copy the virus in large numbers. Usually, this has the incidental effect of killing the cell. I say that it is incidental because the human body has quite a large number of cells and, in most viral infections, the loss of a few cells *is* incidental. Cells divide and replace those that are gone. The problem with HIV is that it continues to kill off particular subsets of your white blood cells—typically CD4 lymphocytes at the rate of more than a billion a day[50]—until the stem cells that replace them are probably exhausted (too old to divide well). As a result, the number of available white blood cells falls suddenly and steeply, the body loses its ability to defend itself, and it dies of infections that would otherwise be trivial. But the destruction of the immune system is far from incidental or trivial.

This sudden decline in the number of white blood cells and the onset of unusual infections defines AIDS. Although HIV attacks other cells, the bulk of the disease results from the immune system's destruction because of the loss of these particular white blood cells.

The virus acts as if it can recognize only mature white blood cells. Stem cells, which produce them, are safe, but every time a cell declares itself a white blood cell—at least a CD4 cell—and enters the general circulation, it is promptly invaded and killed. For a time, often years, the stem cells keep up with the steady loss. A precarious balance is maintained between cell destruction (a billion a day) and cell replacement (a billion new cells a day). The number we measure—CD4 cells in the bloodstream—is a product of the same two opposing forces: production and destruction. But that number is a poor measure both of the work that the stem cells are doing to produce white blood cells and of the virus's destruction of white cells at about the same rate.

It is conceivable that if the rate of destruction increased, we could still measure a normal number of white blood cells circulating in the bloodstream because the production of white blood cells would have increased as well. What we wouldn't see in the measurement is any indication of the frantic cell division or of the frenetic use of metabolic energy needed to wage this war. We wouldn't see this until after several years of infection when the stem cells were finally exhausted: Then the CD4 count would fall dramatically and frighteningly, signaling a death knell through your body, despite every clinical attempt to save you from infection. Unchallenged, infections grow more frequent and more severe, and you die.

And the apparent cause of the stem cell's exhaustion is the telomeric clock running down and stopping stem cell division. Under normal circumstances, stem cells are capable of meeting the demands of most infections during your lifetime, but they are not up to the excessive demand of constant division. This suggests two possible breakthroughs—one for diagnosis, the other for treatment. By measuring the lengths of the telomeres in white blood cells, we might have advance warning of stem cell exhaustion. That might allow us to predict when the immune system will fail, and we might be able to treat the imminent fatal infections before they occur. We have some indication that this early warning is feasible. Some tentative research suggests that the telomeres shorten before clinical changes occur and before the white blood cell counts fall.[51] Following telomere lengths might give us early warning of when an HIV patient will develop AIDS.

Saving the patient's life is another question, which brings up the therapeutic possibility. What if we could reextend the telomeres of the stem cells of the patient with HIV (or with AIDS for that matter)? That wouldn't kill the virus; nor would a renewed ability to produce more white blood cells. It wouldn't even slow the incredible waste of a billion white blood cells a day. However, it *might* prevent stem cell exhaustion, which might resurrect the dying patient. The AIDS patient might become "merely" HIV-positive again, without clinical manifestations, without life-threatening infections, and perhaps without dying from AIDS. Even if nothing else was possible, that possibility alone would justify trying to alter the telomere. For the millions who are dying, for the millions who may yet die, telomere alteration might possibly offer a chance of life. HIV could become a chronic condition, like diabetes, in which the risk of early death is high, but not certain, in which complications are common, but often postponed.

Not only is the evidence for telomeres as clocks strong, but it gives us hope. That hope is for all of us who are aging. It is for children dying of Hutchinson-Gilford syndrome, children who have never yet had a chance to have a normal childhood and who otherwise never will. The hope is for those of us—our neighbors, friends, children, and others—with AIDS, who live with the constant knowledge that an unpleasant death lurks around the corner of tomorrow, or next week, or next year. And, as we will see in Chapter 6, the hope is well-founded; we have already been able to reset the telomere in vitro and we will soon be able to treat many of those diseases caused by short telomeres. But they are not the only diseases that cause suffering and fear, robbing us of our childhood, or our peace, or our integrity. Curiously, the discovery of the mechanism of the telomeric clock also brings hope for diseases such as cancer that have an opposite cause, telomeres that are too long.

DISEASES OF INAPPROPRIATELY LONG TELOMERES

Cancer

We have spoken of cancer already, although not in exactly this context. Cancer is a unique disease that occurs when telomeres relengthen. Because your body expends remarkable effort to ensure that your telomeres will shorten as cells divide, that is what happens in most cases, with almost no exceptions. In fact, only cancer cells manage to evade the shortening once it begins. Moreover, they do not even have especially long telomeres, but they are still too long for the body's health to be maintained. Cancer could be cured if only the telomeres would continue to shorten, as they do in most precancerous cells. So cancer is a disease caused not specifically by long telomeres, but by *inappropriately long* telomeres.

Having already discussed how cancer works in the last chapter, there remains only the question of therapy. Can we alter the telomere length, perhaps by inhibiting the telomerase that cancer cells express, and so cure cancer? As we will see in Chapter 6, we can. Once more, not only is there potential for cure of many of the most serious of human diseases, but the evidence supports our hopes.

ALTERING HUMAN LIFE SPAN

Increasing the average human life span is easy and prosaic. All you have to do is wear your seat belt, exercise, eat carefully (and less), take antioxidant vitamins, avoid smoking, and not antagonize people who carry weapons. All of these are effective means to enhance your average life span, but none of them will alter your maximum potential life span, because they don't have any effect on the limitations imposed by your genetic clock, the telomere. One hundred and twenty years is about the most one can expect to live by being diligent and having an outstanding amount of good luck.

Even so, maximum life span can be altered without telomere alteration. It has been accomplished in nematodes and flies by breeding them for longer lives. Those that live the longest in each generation are chosen as the breeders, while those that die at the usual age have their offspring removed from the breeding pool. In this way, life spans easily double; though as yet this has not been accomplished with humans. In Robert Heinlein's classic *Methuselah's Children*, financial incentive was offered to those whose grandparents were still living to marry one another and have children.[52] Soon their offspring were living longer lives than most of the population. Although in the book the increase in life spans occurred more rapidly than it actually would,[53] the idea is accurate. Theoretically, we could extend the life span of subsequent generations if long-lived people had more children than did others. However, that is unlikely to occur because social constraints and the number of generations required to select for longevity would make success implausible. In addition, it would fly directly in the face of our ethics.

Can we extend the human life span for those of us who are neither worms nor flies and who are not lucky enough to be born into just the right family in Heinlein's fictional world? Human germ cells are ageless, which indicates that some human cells are intrinsically able to avoid aging. We also know that other species can be bred for longer lives, which indicates that nothing is immutable about the normal life span of a multicellular organism. These two examples are evidence that we can alter your cells to extend your maximum life span significantly. Already, scientists have altered the telomere to enable us to turn back and stop the clock.[54] Using normal human fibroblasts, which otherwise reliably age and die in culture, the telomeres have been reextended using telomerase and the telomere end has been "locked" in place to prevent further shortening. Either approach, turning back the clock with telomerase or stopping its countdown with a lock, is effective. In both cases, the result is the same: The cells that were previously destined for senility and death went on dividing and living normally. There was no Hayflick limit for those cells, or what there was was pushed back beyond any semblance of normal aging.

It is important that, if we are to delay or prevent aging, we be able to push back the Hayflick limit, because in species after species, it is directly correlated with the life span.[55] Altering the Hayflick limit, the "life span of a cell," will soon be possible for the whole organism, extending the maximum life span of the entire body. When we can do this not in the laboratory, but in the clinics, we will, perhaps, have conquered aging. Not today, but soon.

CHAPTER 5

TIME RUNS OUT

THE ONLY DISEASE

Old age seems the only disease; all others run into this one.

—RALPH WALDO EMERSON, "CIRCLES"

AGE TOILS PATIENTLY from telomeres to deathbed, picking its way down the paths of our genetic flaws. Emerson was right: One by one, all of our diseases run into this single, final one. Yet old age—the short telomere and the old cell—is also the source of many of our diseases. Whether heart disease, arthritis, or Alzheimer's, aging cells are so much a part of disease that old age might as well be the only disease—causing so many, ending them all. Curiously, we have now come to the point where we can best discuss how aging really works—by discussing disease.

Aging is not merely the result of the actions of free radicals, cells, or telomeres. It is also day-to-day problems, disease, and suffering. Physically, it is weakness, lost memories, aching joints, falling, and brittle, broken bones; or heart disease, shortness of breath, arthritis, cataracts, cancer, and Alzheimer's; it is forgetting your children's names and not being able to walk.

To this point, we have barely strayed from what is known and hardly ventured into the future. It is time to move out of the laboratory and into our lives and into the diseases we live with.

Old age underlies all other diseases as we grow older. The cause of aging is also the cause, or trigger, of most of the diseases of old age. Each has its own unique causes and its own genetic contributions; each is individual and separate from all others. Yet the erosion of the telomere plays a role in all of them—causing one disease directly, hastening another, complicating others. If the telomere did not shorten, most diseases would have a different face; and a few might never appear at all.

How do we go from the loss of our telomeres to the loss of our ability to climb the stairs? How does the crime occur that takes from us first our telomeres, and then our minds and souls? This chapter traces the aging process from the invisible operation of the telomere, to the more manifest behavior of our cells, and finally into the tangible outcomes of decay, discomfort, senility, and death.

IMMORTAL CELLS, MORTAL BODIES

Like one that on a lonesome road
Doth walk in fear and dread,
And having once turned round walks on,
And turns no more his head;
Because he knows a frightful fiend
Doth close behind him tread.

—SAMUEL TAYLOR COLERIDGE, "THE RIME OF
THE ANCIENT MARINER," VI. 10

When biologists talk about cell immortality, they are referring to cells that don't age, not to cells that live forever. After all, even "immortal" cells are still subject to injury and predation; they may be ageless, but they are not actually immortal. And for the same reason, immortality is just as impossible in the organism as a whole. Like cells, even if the organism doesn't age, it will still die. But even having cells that don't age would not guarantee that you won't age. You are not just a collection of cells, ageless or otherwise; you are a collection of *organized* cells. That organization is most important to you: it doesn't matter that much if an individual cell dies and is replaced as long as your body remains intact overall. And while each cell lives, it must function well—not age and fail. You need more than agelessness—you must have ageless cells that respect and maintain the overall organization that is you.

Again, let's consider cancer. If each of your cells were ageless, but cancerous, you would die. Your cells might be "immortal" in the biological sense, but you would still die. Your survival and the survival of all your cells depend on the social behavior of each of your cells. Not only is there no such thing as strict immortality, but to survive, the cells of your body have to do more than just live; they must also continue to fill their social roles. We can, however, aim for an ageless organism. To achieve that, we need both ageless cells and normal cell-to-cell interactions. In other words, we must prevent cell aging without encouraging cancer.

We already know that the life span of an organism correlates with the "life span" of its cells when we grow them in culture (their Hayflick limit). We also know that we can extend that limit in cells—we can make cells ageless in culture. Before we can understand how we will do it in the entire organism, we have to understand not only how cells age, but how the whole body ages. Somehow, we will have to maintain the "social interactions" of our cells, while at the same time turning back the clock that shuts them down. We need to clarify how the shortened telomeres result not only in old cells, but also in an old body—and what other processes, perhaps independent of the telomere, contribute to this. After all, aging is a result of both the telomeric clock and the interactions among cells that go awry when this clock runs down.

CELLS CAUSE HAVOC

Cry "Havoc!" and let slip the dogs of war.

—*Julius Caesar*, III.i

We have already presented an overview of how aging moves from the cells to the entire body. The underlying forces behind aging are the initially balanced and eternal pair of players: entropic damage and our defenses. Aging begins when our defenses are overridden and entropy gains the upper hand.

At the cellular beginning of the aging process, the telomere changes the gene expression in each of your cells. Cell division slows and cells no longer supply the trophic factors—local "hormones," including growth factors, that control the functions, division, and even survival of other cells—required by neighboring cells. No longer is aging confined to just a single cell; now the aging cell is also harming its younger neighbor. Bystander cells, which may still have relatively long telomeres, are stressed by the aging of other cells.

As aging cells begin to affect these bystanders that might otherwise still be "young" and functional, the bystanders, in turn, must alter their own function, to defend themselves against the stress of local inflammation and to take up the load that the aging cell no longer carries. For instance, if the aging cell was responsible for producing insulin, then the cell next to it will now have to produce much more. If the aging cell had the job of dividing and thus reproducing white blood cells, then the cell next to it must now divide more often. If the aging cell held together your arteries, the one next to it will now have twice the stress and twice the work. As these effects—the altering of gene expression and a cell's ability to do its job, the stressing of neighbors, the undermining of organ function—cascade, they are eventually expressed as the diseases we commonly associate with aging.

Those diseases have many contributing causes, however; there is never a simple course from telomere to death. The telomere doesn't simply cause a heart attack or a ruptured aneurysm. Your aorta can rupture because your blood pressure was too high or because your aortic walls were too weak, or for a dozen other reasons, each of which may be partly the result of short telomeres.

Shortening telomeres cause disease, but the route from telomere to disease is complex and influenced by genes, diet, exercise, and luck. Imagine that we knew nothing about strokes, but were trying to understand them. At first glance, all we would see is that the outcome is dramatic and sudden: The person can no longer walk or talk. As decades passed and we did more research, we would realize that what we took for a "stroke" might have been caused either by not enough blood to the brain (narrowed vessels and a clot, for example) or by bleeding within the brain (a vessel that ruptures). We would separate our two types of strokes and name them: infarct or hemorrhage. Looking further at one of these, we would find that the vessel wall was abnormal. Looking deeper, we'd discover that there are characteristic lesions in some of the cells, some of which we'd attribute to hypertension, others to cholesterol, diabetes, viral infection, or trauma. Each understanding of what "causes" stroke could, in turn, be subdivided into smaller parcelings of causation, and each of these could then be subdivided again— until we arrived at the bottom of things. To some extent there is a bottom: The underlying cause of many strokes is the shortening telomere. As we come to understand diseases (whether cancer, stroke, heart attack, or something else), we find more and more contributions from odd and subtle sources, but in many of these, the telomere plays a role.

Heart attacks can be caused by an endless list of contributors, among them cholesterol plaques, electrical problems in your heart, inflammation, stress, lack of exercise, high blood pressure, and smoking. Worse yet, none of these causes is independent; most interact with one another. Cholesterol wouldn't be so bad if you didn't smoke. Smoking would be less dangerous if you didn't have high blood pressure. Blood pressure wouldn't be a problem if your arterial walls weren't injured by a viral infection. And so on.

Heart attacks provide a good example for us, though. The older we grow, the more likely we are to have one. But some people never do, no matter how old they live to be, and others have them in their twenties. Aging alone does not cause heart disease, but it feeds into it through a thousand tributaries. Aging cells contribute to the inflammation that lies at the root of cholesterol plaques; they also change your immune function, the way you process cholesterol, the way your heart paces itself, the strength of your heart muscle, and the way your vessels handle your blood pressure. All of these things, and many more, add to the risk of heart attack, a risk that lies hidden until a single factor reaches its threshold and your heart founders as it tries to beat without enough oxygen and sugar to support itself.

The same is true of other diseases that have become synonymous with growing old. They have dozens, even hundreds, of causes, and aging cells play a role in all of them. Aging is like a series of tributaries, increasing their flow each year, contributing to each disease by adding to its causes. Even without aging you can die of any disease; but aging makes the disease inevitable.

Most people who age at a normal rate can die of heart disease brought on by any number of causes (genes, tobacco, diet, etc.) or by the interactions of several causes. As we grow older, it is more likely that one of those causes will get us. However, with the right genes, the right diet, the right behavior, and a bit of luck, we may never have heart disease at all. In progeric children, the contributions of aging cells are so overwhelming and unavoidable that heart disease occurs even without high cholesterol, smoking, or inactivity. In a normal aging process, aging cells contribute less directly.

Telomere therapy would have no direct effect on smoking, exercise, diet, high cholesterol, or any of the other causes of heart disease. Yet, without the impetus of aging cells and shortening telomeres, your risk of heart disease might remain steady from year to year, instead of climbing as it now does. If cholesterol was accumulating, it would have to accumulate independent of aging. You might still have heart disease, but it would be delayed. The same is true of other diseases that are associated with aging.

The fault lies initially with the cell.

How damaged an individual cell is—how much it contributes to an age-associated disease—is like the worth of a car. It's not just a matter of the odometer reading (or the telomere length in the cell), it is also a matter of how much damage it has. What does it look like and how well does it still run? How you drive your car, where you drive it, and what happens to it—as when another car strikes it at sixty miles an hour—partly determines the worth of your car. At such times, not only

does your car lose value rapidly but you can lose quite a bit yourself—
your life, for example.

Just as the worth of your car is partially determined by external
factors such as road conditions and the driving habits of others, so it
is with your cells. Even a new car isn't worth much if it has had salt
damage and two major collisions; a neuron with a long telomere isn't
worth much with aging vessels and faulty glial cells around it. The
more other cells injure them, the faster even young cells lose value
and contribute to disease. Using the car analogy again, it's as though
every time another car hits yours, the odometer reading increases two
thousand miles. Some cells are damaged by their neighbors; others are
forced to divide when cells are lost.

Cell division is not random. Your cells divide, or don't, in response
to dozens of simultaneous and usually conflicting signals from other
cells. These external signals have a lot to do with how often the cell
divides and thus how fast the telomeric clock runs down. Each cell
takes in the information from other cells, considers it in light of its
own circumstances, and then divides, or doesn't divide. The skin cells
on the back of your hand divide not only in response to their own
internal readiness—or whims?—but also to signals from neighboring
cells and hormones from cells several feet away. Aging can be determined by, and is best measured by, the telomere, but the *rate* of aging
is determined by the needs of other cells, urging a cell to divide or
pleading with it not to; from this standpoint, aging is the result of
interactions with other cells, not just the shortening telomere.

There is a second sense in which aging is the result of other cells.
Young, healthy cells that are capable of dividing can be made to age
faster, when they are damaged by other, older cells. An aging cell
might no longer support a younger, healthy one that depends upon it;
the younger cell might require some protein or other molecule normally made by the older, failing cell; or an aging cell might injure
another, younger cell by inflammation or release of toxins (from the
innocent cell's perspective, it is injury not aging, although it can accelerate aging). If the younger cell responds by dividing repeatedly, its
telomere will shorten and it will age further. For example, if a skin
cell gets too old to divide, its neighboring, "younger" cells will be
forced to divide faster to produce enough skin cells. Their telomeres

will shorten, resulting in their aging more rapidly than before. Thus, an aging cell can force other cells to accelerate their own aging.

On the other hand, if an aging, dividing cell merely injures a younger, *nondividing* cell, the result is still merely injury, not aging. If a glial cell, becoming old, no longer supports the neurons around it or, worse, causes inflammation and damages them, it causes an injury, but not aging. Unlike skin cells, the neuron's response isn't to divide and so it doesn't shorten its telomeres any faster than it did before. However, it does fail; it stops working and so do the circuits that it is part of. The injured neuron no longer responds to signals from other neurons; it does not signal back to them, and it may even withdraw some of its contacts. Even if it doesn't "age," the brain's function has been diminished.

As we examine aging at more clinical and personal levels, we see that it involves much more than the telomeres running out. If neurons die because glial cells have lost their telomeres, the result may be Alzheimer's disease. Is that aging? From the sufferer's perspective, it certainly is. The neurons may not have aged, but the glial cells did and that was enough to trigger the disease.

Thus, aging and the diseases we associate with it involve more than which cells have short telomeres and which do not. Aging begins with the telomeres but does not end there. It is a process that creeps through your body, sometimes in the guise of aging cells, sometimes in the role of bystanders that are pulled down along with them. It infiltrates your tissues, subverts your systems, and catches you unawares.

A CELL'S WORTH

The worth of a state, in the long run, is the worth of the individuals composing it.

—JOHN STUART MILL, *ON LIBERTY*

The worth of any group of cells is the worth of the cells composing it. Whether the group is a tissue (muscle, skin, or nerve, for example), an organ (heart, liver, or brain), or a system (cardiovascular, gastro-intestinal, or immune system), the function of the whole is determined by the individual cells that it is made up of and by the relationship of those cells. Those cells and their relationship change with age, varying only in how they show it. Some groups of cells barely change with age; others show catastrophic changes. Some remain relatively healthy; others become obviously diseased. Aging feeds into all of these changes, from the subtle alteration to overt disease. The diseases vary, as does the suffering we endure. In some of us the heart ages faster and fails first; in others it's the brain, the kidneys, or the lungs. All of our organs age to varying degrees and each of us differs in how fast we age.

As we understand better how each organ ages, we will also learn which changes caused by aging—and which diseases—we can reverse or prevent. We will almost certainly be able to prevent heart disease and probably Alzheimer's disease, but will not be able to reverse their consequences. However, we will be able to reverse the aging damage to the vessels that cause heart disease, the aging of the glial cells that might lie at the root of Alzheimer's disease, and the aging of other groups of cells that are the source of clinical aging. To understand what we can prevent and what we can reverse, we need to know how age-related diseases grow from these aging groups of cells.

BLOOD VESSELS

If the blood vessels, which support all other cells, fail, then the cells in every tissue organ, or system they supply will fail as well. And because those vessels do fail as we get older, they lie at the root of the apparent aging of many other groups of cells.[1] For example, most of the "aging" of our hearts is not cardiac aging, but vessel aging, and to a remarkable but lesser extent, the same is true of the aging brain. Many age-related diseases of the brain—strokes are a good example—are caused by aging of the brain's blood vessels.

The structure of a blood vessel varies with its size and whether it is an artery or a vein. The arrangement is always a tube made of cells in several, concentric layers—only two or three of which matter to us here. The innermost, endothelial, cells are similar in many ways to skin cells, such as fibroblasts: They line the blood vessels, divide and replace lost endothelial wall cells, and slow down and change—i.e., age—when they have divided too many times. Any time one of these cells dies due to injury by high blood pressure, cholesterol, inflammation, or the stress of blood flow especially where your vessels branch, it is replaced by neighboring cells that divide to fill the gap; the neighboring cells' telomeres shorten with each division until they can no longer keep up with the need for replacement cells.

If the next layer is exposed—if only transiently—it allows more inflammation, growth of the smooth muscle cells of the vessel wall (especially if they have certain viral infections), and deposition of cholesterol. The vessel wall narrows and becomes scarred, irregular, and sticky; all of this contributes to more stress on the cells lining the vessel. Blood tries to pass through a narrower, irregular vessel; turbulence and shear stress increase; more cells lining the vessel die; and the cycle continues and worsens.

As the endothelial cells age, they also slow their production of "trophic factors" (local "hormones" made by cells in one tissue which affect the function of and are often required for the survival of cells in a neighboring tissue), which changes cell function in deeper layers of the vessel wall. Loss of these factors causes clots to adhere more easily, smooth muscle cells to proliferate, white cells to invade, cholesterol to accumulate, and a host of other changes to occur, all of which are part of plaque formation and vessel disease.[2]

Cells age fastest in the parts of your vessels that are most stressed. Those are the sites where telomeres are shortest and where the cells are slow to divide and unable to produce normal amounts of trophic factors for neighboring cells. Those same sites, where the telomeres are shortest, are where aneurysms and cholesterol plaques are most frequent. High blood pressure, high cholesterol, diabetes, and smoking all play a role in vessel disease by stressing the vessels—thereby accelerating cellular aging—and by causing further damage to other neighboring cells as the endothelial cells age and cause secondary changes in these other cells.

This same general plot can continue even without a few of the major players. Progerics, for example, don't have the same cholesterol deposition that most of us will have in old, or even middle, age and yet they still have damage to their blood vessels and still go on to die of heart disease and strokes. Even if we subtract cholesterol, high blood pressure, and inflammation from the equation, vessel disease can still occur. But with all of these players on stage and cellular aging as the main character, the drama becomes a short and fast-paced tragedy.

Aging causes disease in the major vessels, such as the aorta, the coronary arteries, and the cerebral arteries, when telomere loss no longer allows the cells lining the blood vessels to replace lost cells and plaque is permitted to form in the vessel wall. The process accelerates aging in any nearby cell capable of division and injures nearby cells, capable of division or not. The aging of cells in vessel walls is responsible for most of the pathology that occurs in aging vessels.[3]

At the other end of the size spectrum from the aorta and other large vessels are the capillaries—the smallest and most important vessels. They deliver most of the blood's oxygen and nutrients and take away most of the carbon dioxide and waste your cells toss out. Unlike larger vessels, they regrow wherever surrounding tissue is injured. However slight the injury, capillary beds are likely to be damaged and they must be replaced.

As their telomeres tick down, cell replacement fails and with it the body's ability to maintain healthy capillaries. And as *those* fail, so does the rest of your body. The capillaries begin to leak, no longer extend to as many places, and no longer grow as well. Cells that relied upon a high-quality distribution system must make do with nutrients and oxygen diffusing from a distance. Proteins, other molecules, and invaders that kept within the vessels now find easier access to places they don't belong.

The aging of capillaries resembles that of large vessels in its slower division of cells. Whether capillary aging, like large-vessel aging, is also marked by loss of trophic factors and the attendant pathology is not known. Aging capillaries, however, are clearly different in another way: They act like control valves in some respects, and the flexibility of that control diminishes with age.

Capillaries aren't passive: They shrink and expand in response to the needs of the cells around them. As the capillary cells age, their actions are slower and less effective. At rest, the muscle in a sixty-year-old may have the same excellent blood supply as in a twenty-year-old, but should that muscle begin to exercise, the sixty-year-old's capillaries will no longer provide what the muscle demands.

This active response to tissue needs is one way in which your body adapts as you exercise—or even as you stand up in the morning. As you age, these responses become less reliable, ultimately leading to high blood pressure. Both smaller and larger vessels are crucial to maintaining a normal blood pressure. Although larger vessels cannot constrict and open, as can capillaries, their elasticity serves the same purpose and it decreases with age. Collagen that provides strength and elastin that provides flexibility no longer turn over as fast as they did when you were young and there is greater cross-linking of collagen molecules. The combination of aging capillary beds, which are less responsive, and aging large vessels, which are stiffer, results in higher blood pressure and with it more stress on the cells lining the vessels. Hypertension is both a cause and an effect of aging cells in your blood vessels.

The correspondence between aging and high blood pressure is so striking that aging has been called "muted hypertension" and hypertension "accelerated aging."[4] Despite the correlation, neither description is really accurate. Like heart disease and most other diseases related to aging, hypertension is a disease having many causes, the effects of almost all of them enhanced by aging as your cells divide. Aging isn't synonymous with hypertension, but as the telomeres disappear blood pressure can rise in a slow but vicious cycle. And as that happens, as capillaries are lost, as vessels narrow, as peripheral cells cry out for a better blood supply, as the blood pressure rises, and as aneurysms appear, something finally fails: perhaps your brain, or your kidneys, or your heart.

THE HEART

The heart doesn't age much, perhaps because most of its cells don't divide much. The clocks of those cells are still fully wound. Yet when we think of aging, we conjure up pictures of heart attacks and congestive heart failure; of weak hearts, bad hearts, and old hearts. Most of the aging of the heart is due to the deterioration of vessels that supply the heart and the rest of your body.[5] As you age, your heart is asked to do more and is paid less for it. As the vessels age, the blood pressure rises and your heart works harder. As the coronary vessels that supply the heart age, the heart muscle receives less blood. More work, less pay. When these two trends cross each other, the heart fails, often dramatically. Even if only one vessel becomes too narrow to supply the blood, and its oxygen, to the heart muscle, the muscle dies; the pump fails, the heart stops, the body dies. Even in less dramatic circumstances, the outcome is cumulative and poor. The heart loses small portions of its muscle, its output falls, and the body is no longer capable of what it once was.

There are primary heart diseases—viral myocarditis and congenital malformations, for instance—and secondary, garden-variety ones—such as myocardial infarctions and rhythm disturbances—which result from aging of cells in the vessels. Primary heart disease is rare—but what about primary aging of the heart? Does the heart age independently of its aging vessels? It has fibroblasts that divide and age, like most other tissues; those cells age, but they are in the minority. The heart *muscle* cells probably also age, but we don't know much about the process yet. Clearly the muscle cells accumulate age pigments as they grow older—to the point where in old age 30 percent of the heart's weight may be lipofuscin. But we still don't know whether that is because of aging vessels (making it harder for the cells to break down and oxidize their wastes) or simply an unavoidable accumulation of waste (no matter how good the vessels were). Heart cells may be damaged because of aging in the vessels (secondary aging) or because of some degree of primary aging in the heart cells as well.

Although cellular aging can be reversed with telomere therapy, once the cells of the heart are gone, they cannot be replaced by alterations to your telomeres. If the heart (and all of its cells) is merely suffering from the aging of its vessels, however, with no irreversible change as yet, then telomere therapy promises to reverse the trend before it is too late.

THE BRAIN

Most people regard the brain as the body's most important collection of cells, since it represents the most essential part of ourselves—our minds and personalities. The estimated 100 billion or more cells in your brain is where you live in a very personal fashion. It's where your personality, memories, and soul are found. And here, in a fragile quart and a half of jelly, is where aging often becomes tragedy; here we lose ourselves. Although heart disease makes up a large percentage of the ailments experienced as our days draw to a close, Alzheimer's disease and the other dementias represent our worst nightmares of what the evenings of our lives can be.

The body's nervous system is composed of the brain and a host of peripheral nerves. Neurons account for only 10 percent of the cells, the other 90 percent being glial cells, on which the neurons depend; far more is known about neurons than about glial cells, the "other cells" of the nervous system. Among the functions of the glial cells is the careful maintenance of the chemical environment around neurons. In addition, they remove extra neural transmitters, and respond to them; regulate nutrients; determine blood flow; and generally make sure that neurons are pampered in a carefully controlled and constant environment. They allow no surprises, famine, or unpleasantness to attach to the neurons. Without these careful housekeepers, neurons would become undependable and would soon be damaged. Neurons die when excitatory neural transmitters such as glutamate aren't rapidly mopped up by glial cells.[6] They die without trophic factors[7] that glial cells produce and supply to neurons.[8] The glial cells allow neurons to do what they do so miraculously.

The diseases we associate with the nervous system—strokes, Alzheimer's, and other dementias—occur because the glia, unlike the neurons that they protect, age and die. And we become susceptible to them because our blood vessels "age" as do our glial cells. As with the heart, it is not so much the nervous system per se that ages as the vessels and the cells—the glia—that aren't neurons at all. The glia age, whereas neurons do not.

The problem of aging vessels is not specific to the nervous system, although—just as with cells in the heart and in contrast to most other cells in the body—neurons die almost immediately when the vessels fail. The damage from a few minutes of lost circulation can never be canceled by years of normal blood flow afterward. Vessels clog and we have strokes; they burst and we have bleeding in the brain—and in both cases we are never the same, either because we lost great numbers of neurons or because we lost our lives. Aging vessels result in aging diseases affecting our nervous systems.

But aging vessels account for only a third of brain aging.[9] The majority of dementias may be caused by aging glial cells. Glial cells continue to divide throughout life, slowly shortening their telomeres.[10] Why are they replaced when neurons are not?[11] Glial cells are frequently injured, lost, and replaced; there are no irreplaceable glial cells. Glia, roughly speaking, are generic, but neurons are not.[12] Each neuron has specific, often distant connections that define what you can do, how you can do it, and who you are.

As your vessels age, the glial cells are replaced; the remaining glial cells divide, their telomeres shorten, the glial cells age, and they finally fail in their sole job of supporting and pampering neurons; the neurons then die and *cannot* be replaced. Your glia age, your neurons die, your abilities fade. The nervous system ages.

Alzheimer's disease doesn't work that simply. But then, neither does heart disease, nor any other age-related disease. In all of these diseases, including Alzheimer's, aging cells and eroding telomeres play a decisive and often primary role. Without aging glial cells you might still succumb to Alzheimer's; without aging cells in the walls of your vessels you might still acquire arteriosclerosis; but without aging cells and shortened telomeres, the process would probably take far longer, be more dependent on other genetic influences, and in some of us never occur at all. Alzheimer's disease is a complex disorder that is not understood, but aging cells and lost telomeres may lie at its heart. Dementias, particularly Alzheimer's, may turn out to be intimately related to the glial cells: Their inflammation,[13] their trophic factors,[14] and their cellular aging may prove to be responsible for the loss of neurons and that loss of function that we fear the most.

Telomere therapy will avert strokes and perhaps Alzheimer's disease. Reversing aging in the vessels, we can prevent but not reverse strokes; we can prevent the death of neurons but not replace them once lost. In Alzheimer's, however, more than anywhere else, there is so much yet unknown. Alzheimer's disease and the other dementias—while complex and strongly affected by other, especially genetic, factors—are probably even more strongly abetted by shortening telomeres in aging cells and to that extent they will be preventable.

THE SKIN

The skin is the organ that ages most obviously. With one glance we estimate age and with often imprudent, and impudent, accuracy. Aged

skin with its liver spots, wrinkles, thinness, and poor healing is common
and obvious. The very fact that your skin is so exposed in public is
one reason it ages: The sun and day-to-day trauma accelerate its aging
by damaging and killing cells. To keep up with their losses, skin cells
respond by dividing quickly. Their rapid division means that more cells
reach their Hayflick limits; and old skin has fewer cells and the ones
that remain are shoddy workers.

The pool of cells becomes smaller not only because old cells can't
divide as fast as they once did, but also because cells are more readily
lost as you age. The turnover rate becomes half of what it was when
you were younger, and you lose cells faster because they are less protected and less supported. The decrease in pool size is true of all the
cells that make up your skin, not just fibroblasts. The number of blood
vessels in the skin decreases as you age, so they provide poorer nutrition. The body's temperature control begins to limp as the skin's capillaries no longer open and close as readily to adjust our temperature.
We overheat easily, we chill easily. There are fewer immune cells in
the skin, and the ones there are are less effective, diminishing their
protection, leaving bacteria, viruses, and fungi a free rein to infect and
kill more cells. Nerves have fewer branches, so your response to pain
slows and becomes erratic. You incur more damage because you are
no longer as aware of danger. You have fewer fat cells, so your insula-
tion from the cold and your cushion against trauma weaken. Owing to
the reduction in pigment cells, your hair becomes white and, more
important, ultraviolet light now penetrates farther and damages more
of your cells as you age. Fewer sweat glands leave you less able to
release heat by evaporation; fewer oil glands leave your skin dry and
less protected from damage and infection.

All of these cell losses contribute to a harsher life for the ones that
remain. As the rate of damage increases, the need for new cells accelerates. Unfortunately, the shortened telomeres have a great deal of trouble meeting that need. When you are young, your skin is held firmly
together in a convoluted middle layer, but as you age and your cells
die off, this junction simplifies to an almost tablelike flatness, until the
bonds between cells break with the slightest stress. In thin sheets, your
skin tears away with an innocent fall, healing slowly or not at all. No
matter what the danger—trauma, cold, infection, or radiation—as the

number of skin cells decreases with age, the risk to the rest of the body increases disproportionately.

In addition, the cells that remain don't work as well. For example, pigment cells not only grow fewer, but are poor at making melanin and controlling their growth. They often multiply into small patches, liver spots, that are a hallmark of aging.

Old cells respond slowly and inaccurately to signals from other cells; especially those in glands and vessels. Skin cells are poorer at making vitamin D; collagen and elastin production is slower and turnover slows down. Within the old cell, turnover slows and damaged proteins accumulate. Outside the cell, damage accumulates in the proteins—collagen and elastin—that lie between cells. They are too old to divide and replace missing cells, and too old to produce and replace damaged proteins.

As long as the cells that remain are representative of all your normal cell types—as long as you haven't killed off all of your gland cells, for example—these changes are reversible. Once we can extend the telomeres of these cells, missing skin cells could be replaced and protein turnover increased again. Most of the aging that occurs in your skin is not only preventable, but reversible.

THE GASTROINTESTINAL SYSTEM

The cells of your intestines depend on cell division, in the same way that skin cells and those lining your vessel walls do. The lining of your intestine is replaced entirely every two to five days.[15] To keep up with this quick turnover, the cells must divide rapidly. As a result, the lining, and the other layers of the intestine, becomes thinner and less effective as you age.[16] The outer intestinal wall weakens, leading to diverticular disease as little "pockets" of intestine balloon out from the wall and threaten to rupture. Glands become fewer and those remaining secrete less. This is true of the salivary glands in your mouth, the secretory glands of your stomach, as well as glands secreting a host of substances in your intestines; in almost all of them, the number of cells decreases as does their output. Food absorption becomes more erratic; certain vitamins (D, for instance) and some minerals (calcium and perhaps iron) are less well absorbed as we age.

Even so, the gastrointestinal system doesn't age nearly as much as we expect it to. Given the high cellular division rate and our knowledge of the limits imposed by the telomeric clock, we might expect it to fall apart—and you with it. The fact that it does so well in old age is probably due more to its remarkable redundancy than to any lack of changes resulting from aging.[17] The changes that do occur are likely due both to the direct aging of those cells that make up your gastro-intestinal walls and to the indirect effects of aging in the blood vessels that supply those walls. These vessels can accumulate cholesterol plaques and all the other hallmarks of vascular disease, even a form of "intestinal angina." And all of these aging changes, like those due to cells and vessels that have aged elsewhere in your body, can be reversed if we can use telomere therapy before the cells are lost.

THE KIDNEYS

The kidneys shrink and fail to filter blood as they age. The initial portion of the filtration system—the glomeruli—has the most tissue loss as you age, and what remains is increasingly dysfunctional. As the kidney's blood vessels age, not only do they provide less blood to cells that need it, but they are also prone to short-circuit the filtration apparatus altogether and return unfiltered blood to the body. All this renders the kidney less and less able to do its job. Most of the aging of the kidney is probably secondary to vessel aging[18] and so is reversible. If part of the problem is that older kidney cells have divided and are nearing the ends of their telomeres, then that too will be reversible by telomere therapy. But to the extent that aging causes permanent loss of the complex structures that filter, refilter, and adjust the blood chemistry, we will only be able to prevent—and not reverse—aging in the kidney.

THE LUNGS

The lungs age more because of what you do to them than because of what the years do. But even without tobacco and pollution, lungs still age reliably and continually, mostly owing to changes in the connective tissues of the lung. With age—just as in the skin—the turnover of collagen and elastin slows down, damage accumulates, and connective tissue becomes weaker and less flexible. Your chest wall becomes stiffer and it requires more effort for you to breathe. The smallest parts of your lungs—the alveoli or air sacs, in which you actually absorb oxygen and get rid of carbon dioxide—are less elastic and more likely to collapse. You work harder to breathe and get less return for the effort. As with the skin, fibroblasts are the source of these connective tissue changes, and they divide and replace missing cells.

Unlike the fibroblasts of the skin, damage is not the result of trauma and ultraviolet exposure. Damage still occurs and cells are lost as you get older, but in the lungs, the fibroblasts are injured by pollution and damaged by the oxygen they must face without the protection your other cells have. Your skin, for instance, has an outermost layer of dead cells, like the bark of a tree. Most of your body's cells receive oxygen only in small amounts, meted out by your red blood cells. Even your mouth and throat have the slight protection of a thin mucous layer. However, your lung cells lack even this scant protection: they must take the brunt of this damage while performing their job—transferring oxygen in and carbon dioxide out.

Oxygen is vital in small amounts; in large amounts it kills cells, especially fibroblasts in your lungs. As they are replaced, the telomeric clocks in the remaining cells that divide to produce them wind down. As the telomeres shorten, the cells become less effective and less able to continue dividing. As you age, fewer of your lung cells are replaced; the spongy mass of your lung comes to have less sponge and more air; the air sacs grow larger and simpler—and as they grow simpler, you become less able to move oxygen from the air into your blood. All of us experience this problem at least to a small degree, but in some the lungs have become mere shadows of their younger selves. Less capable and less efficient, they lose the reserve that allows us to run, to go upstairs, and, finally, simply to walk. By the time we are in our sixties, most of us notice only that we can no longer run as well or for as long. But for others of us, those who smoke or are simply unlucky, the loss comes early and is crippling.

Replacing telomeres will never make up for the damage we inflict on ourselves: There is no substitute for caring for your body. The delicate and complex structure of alveoli, once lost, cannot be rebuilt.

Yet with telomere therapy we may be able to maintain your lungs indefinitely in the day-to-day campaign against oxygen—the necessary enemy.

THE MUSCULOSKELETAL SYSTEM: JOINTS, BONES, MUSCLES

Our joints hurt, our bones break, our muscles weaken. In each case, aging occurs, but for slightly different reasons. Your joints are made of cartilage, which breaks down with age. This breakdown results from cellular aging, trauma, and your genes. The degree of trauma and the particular genes that were employed in building you determine how fast your cells age: This is especially true of the cartilage that lines your joints, receiving every jolt, push, and step. If you spend your days jogging, the cartilage of your knees ages faster. If your genes are up to the challenge, you may continue to jog into your nineties; if not, you may find yourself creaking in your twenties.

As telomeres shorten, these cells become less able to produce and replace cartilage proteins and they become less able to divide and replace cells lost to the crush and squeeze of daily life in your joints. As in vessel disease—where even without aging, cholesterol and high blood pressure bring about a slow death—repetitive trauma will injure the cells of your joints. Also as in your vessels, aging brings on arthritis that would otherwise be delayed or never seen at all. If you treat your joints well and reset the aging clock in the cells that line your joints, they may last indefinitely.

Your bones are continually being recycled. One type of cell, osteoblasts, makes bone; and another, osteoclasts, destroys it. Those two cell types are in a wavering balance, as they continually remodel your bones. Together they determine the size of the total pool of bone in your body. If bone-forming cells prevail, as they do while you are growing, you gain bone mass; if bone-destroying cells prevail as they do in osteoporosis, you lose bone mass.

While the balance is important, so is the overall rate of turnover. Fast turnover means faster healing, but wasted energy; slow turnover conserves cellular energy, but slows healing. In old age, your bones don't heal well and they break easily. In your youth, if you fall while skiing at high speed, you may break your leg, but it takes considerable force to fracture a bone and then it heals quickly. However, in old age, if you stumble and fall to the carpet, even gently, you might break your hip; it takes almost no force and heals slowly and even then perhaps never perfectly.

In old age, you have fewer bone-forming cells. That alone would be enough to slow turnover and account for osteoporosis and poorer healing. Unfortunately, you also absorb less calcium (particularly over the age of seventy), exercise less (which discourages your bone formation and turnover), and have less estrogen (if you are a woman). Estrogen slows bone reabsorption. Estrogen loss, after menopause, is like taking the brake off bone loss; bone destruction moves into high gear, bone formation has been slowing with age, and the pool of total bone falls imperceptibly, but steadily.

Your bones are like the house in which we pull out one more nail every day: Everything appears to be in order until the wind blows. When you're thirty, you have to fall twenty feet out of a tree to break your vertebra; when you're seventy, you need only sit in the couch and cough to make the same vertebra collapse. They even begin to collapse gradually of their own weight, shrinking and wedging into ill-defined shadows on X rays, your height lost, your back bent, your bones evaporating within you.

We could reset the telomeres of stem cells that make your bone-forming cells, but the high rate of bone destruction is probably related to estrogen, and other factors. Even if telomere therapy enhances bone formation, estrogen supplements may still be needed.[19]

Your muscles don't actually age so much as suffer from disuse and aging vessels. The disuse is understandable. You tire easily because your heart and lungs have to work harder. Your muscles also suffer from the sins of aging in other systems. As your chest wall stiffens, it takes more muscle work to move your ribs. As your ligaments lose elasticity, your muscles are forced to do a job that was previously done for free. As your lungs lose cells, you have to breathe harder to absorb the same amount of oxygen. Despite having to work harder, the muscles are paid less. As the vessels age and the capillary bed shrinks, the muscles have a harder and harder time acquiring the nutrients and oxygen that allow them to do the increased amount of work you ask of them.

THE ENDOCRINE SYSTEMS

The endocrine systems have long been accused of being the source of aging. The accusation is largely, but not completely, false. Estrogen cycles, for example, appear to have a clock that is independent of cellular aging; they are controlled by your total lifetime estrogen exposure rather than by shortening telomeres.

The endocrine systems include insulin, the thyroid hormones, the steroid hormones, growth hormone, and a host of others. Some hormones decrease with age; others are found in the same concentrations in spite of aging, but their turnover is slowed.[20] Your response to hormones is often blunted as you age: sometimes because the hormone receptors are less numerous, often for other, unknown reasons.

Response times are slower for insulin also. Usually, when your blood sugar rises, your body produces more insulin; the same thing happens when you age, but your response is delayed and less accurate. The cells become less efficient in responding to insulin. Insulin is produced and the cells receive the message, "take up sugar," but the response is lackadaisical.

Thyroid hormones—along with several dozen other factors—determine the rate of your metabolism and their levels become less reliable with age.[21] The brain becomes less accurate in overseeing thyroid function, the cells of your body respond abnormally, and your immune system grows sloppy as you age.

Steroid hormones divide naturally into two major groups: sexual steroids, such as estrogen and testosterone, which regulate sexual function; and adrenal steroids, which regulate your carbohydrate, protein, mineral, and water metabolism.[22] Steroid hormones directly affect gene expression, but we do not yet know to what extent this is changed by aging. Although steroid hormones maintain steady blood levels as you age, sexual steroids decrease.

The decline in sexual steroids follows differing patterns for women and men. The pattern for women, is cyclical and reliable until they near menopause, then the system stutters and their steroid levels fall dramatically. We still do not know to what extent menopause is timed by a telomeric clock, but the onset most likely results from the loss of ova; menopausal women have few, or no, ova left.[23] Although women begin life with far more ova than will be used to prepare monthly eggs, they lose an increasing number with each ovulation, until by menopause none are left.

The most common beliefs for the causes of menopause are either that it is the result of lost ova, or that it is caused by accumulated estrogen exposure. It is known that a woman loses ova each month, and more and more with successive menses, until there are no more ova and her menses stop. But it is equally clear that there are some cells in the brain or ovary, or both, that "count" up her total estrogen exposure and stop her menses when some cutoff point is reached in midlife. Neither of these theories attributes menopause to aging or to aging cells.

But aging cells might still play a role. The cells around each ova might divide, age, and change over the years, becoming less able to support and care for the ova. That could explain why, as a woman ages, her rate of ova loss increases. In such a case, aging cells would, indirectly, be playing a role in menopause. The same might also be true of cells that "count" estrogen exposure; those cells might divide, in the ovary, or be supported by cells that divide in the brain. If the menopausal clock is, even distantly, influenced by cells that divide—and whose telomeres therefore shorten—then telomere therapy could delay menopause.

The loss of sexual steroids in men is generally thought to be due to aging cells in the testes, and to be a slow, constant decline from young adulthood to old age. Although here again, there is much that is not known, the system appears unlikely to have any additional, complex clock timing the decrease in function. More likely, the decline parallels normal cellular aging, in either the capillaries or the supportive cells within the testes, and so would be reversible.

Another sexual steroid, dehydroepiandrosterone—or DHEA—has intrigued researchers of aging for thirty years.[24] DHEA is the most common steroid in your blood. Its levels decline with age in a fairly linear fashion, its function is unclear, and its congenital absence is apparently fatal. Some strains of rats given DHEA live longer, but not always. Although the few facts we have are tantalizing,[25] most likely the decrease of DHEA with age is secondary to aging in the adrenal gland, which makes most of our DHEA. If DHEA were the primary cause of aging, we might expect to find abnormal adrenal function in progerics and we don't.

The adrenal glands are also critical for your response to stress. Robert Sapolsky, a professor at Stanford University, argues that every time you experience stress, you lose certain brain cells and with them memory.[26] When you are stressed—which causes you to release steroids from your adrenal gland—you risk losing neurons that are needed for your memory. Any additional stress, such as not enough oxygen, insufficient blood sugar, poor blood flow, etc., kills more neurons critical to memory. With accumulated stress, not only do you lose memory function, but you also lose the ability to turn off the steroid that is causing the damage, which increases the rate of damage. With every additional stress things get worse; more neurons are lost, and dementia progresses.

The neurons do not die because of adrenal steroids by themselves; they die when some additional stress occurs. Do those neurons die because, after stress has forced them to the edge of the cliff, vessel disease, and hence shortening telomeres, pushes them over? Do the aging and the damaged vessels of your brain allow stress to become dementia, when otherwise it would remain merely stress? Or perhaps the neurons die because the glial cells that surround them have aged and are no longer able to buffer the dangers when the neurons are stressed. If Sapolsky is right about stress, what will happen when we reset the cellular clocks of aging? We don't know. There remains room for optimism, but this may become another example of "final aging": a process that, like others we must discuss in Chapter 7, cannot be turned back or perhaps altered at all.

The hormone most often said to affect aging is growth hormone. It plays a pivotal but "intermediate" role in the aging process. The lack of this hormone doesn't bring about aging, but rather the hormone lies in the middle of the aging cascade. Giving supplemental growth hormone to the aging body will restore some lost muscle mass and redistribute your fat, but it will not affect many other common aging changes—and additional growth hormone causes more serious problems, such as diabetes. The hormone, like many others, is produced by the pituitary gland at the base of the brain. We still don't know why these brain cells slow their production of growth hormone as you age; all we know is that they become less responsive to signals from the brain, secreting less and less growth hormone. The pattern of decline mimics that of the sexual steroids: It falls gradually and steadily in men, but not until menopause in women.[27]

Once again, telomere therapy should be able to reverse the aspects of this decline that result from shortening telomeres in glial cells.

Melatonin, a hormone secreted by the pineal gland at the top of your brain stem, has also recently been implicated in aging.[28] Like DHEA, its levels decline with age and, like DHEA, a daily supplement of melatonin may help slow some of the clinical problems of aging, but it does not reset the cellular clocks of aging that are responsible for these problems, nor can it extend the maximum life span.[29]

THE IMMUNE SYSTEM

Your immune system is your body's police force and judiciary. It consists largely of cells with long memories that recall which cells are your responsible citizens and which are invaders; they know whether the offenders are viruses, bacteria, parasites, or cancer cells (the sociopaths of your body). The immune cells find the criminals, pass judgment, and implement an immediate death sentence. The essence of immune function is to correctly and quickly distinguish friend from foe. Leaving normal cells in peace is just as important as attacking abnormal ones and invaders. As we age, our immune system fails at both of these responsibilities. It becomes more likely to attack your healthy cells and less likely to attack cancers and invading organisms. It becomes sloppy and slow, and its memory fails.

This failure of your police force is partly due to having fewer officers on the beat—for example, the number of immune cells in your skin declines. It is also partly due to their deficient "training": For both reasons fewer T lymphocytes are mature and functional in old age.[30] Again, as with other cells, this decrease most likely occurs because shortened telomeres prevent cell division and replacement. The poorer functioning of these aging cells results from altered gene expression that occurs as those same telomeres approach complete erosion. And both the ability to divide and the ability to function normally may be amenable to telomere therapy.

Reversal of aging in the immune system will solve multiple problems, and may even solve problems we do not yet attribute to immune system aging. Failure of the older immune system leads to a higher rate of death from infections that merely annoy the young and middle-aged; these include pneumonias, as well as cellulitis, influenza, and dozens of others.

In aging every failing component increases the likelihood of another failure elsewhere, and this is especially true of the immune system. The changes caused by aging in your lungs increase the chances that you will contract pneumonia, while the aging of your immune system increases the odds that you will die of it. The aging of your blood vessels makes it more difficult for your immune system to locate and kill bacteria; your thinner skin improves the opportunity for bacteria to enter in the first place. Your aging nervous system contributes to the likelihood that you will fall and cut your skin, and that bacteria will enter more easily.

An aging immune system alone would create problems in fighting infection; but an aging immune system together with an aging body sharply diminish your chances of survival. Not only does your body fail to attack external invaders, but it will have trouble with its internal enemies as well. The immune system is responsible for destroying cancer cells; it does that job so well that you remain unaware of the majority of malignant cells that would otherwise kill you. Unfortunately, this monitoring falters as you age. Not only do the number of cancer cells increase in middle age, but also your ability to recognize and kill them. At the same time, your cells are not as good at repairing your DNA—and it is DNA errors that lie at the heart of cancer. In short, you have more cancer cells and you aren't as efficient at destroying them. Clinically, the result is that cancer occurs more frequently as we age, as does death due to cancer. If we could reverse this situation, we would significantly reduce the lethality of cancer.

Equally disastrous is the problem of mistaking your healthy cells for the enemy. Autoimmune disease, in which your immune system attacks your own normal cells, increases with age. Scleroderma, rheumatoid arthritis, lupus, and dozens of other disorders, result from an immune system run amok. Yet the fault may not lie only in the aging immune system.

Though the immune system becomes myopic with age, the cells it attacks also alter as they age. Your joints are attacked, but that is partly the result of infection, trauma, and poor circulation, which are the effects of aging cells in your blood vessels, in the joint cartilage, and in the ligaments that should maintain a taut alignment. All of these factors have been implicated in the damage that occurs in aging joints; all can be blamed on aging telomeres, and all encourage the immune system to attack the joint surface.

AIDS, although not a disease of aging at all, might be considered a disease in which a small, but crucial part of the immune system, CD4 cells, are induced to age (by dividing) rapidly by HIV, the virus that causes AIDS. To a less dramatic extent, what happens to CD4 cells in AIDS occurs to the rest of your immune system during normal aging.

As you age, not only do you have fewer officers, with poorer training, but the citizens of your body's community are ruder. The criminals increase daily, and social problems abound in every community of your body, at every level of investigation. The body's government asks more of its citizens and gives less; resources diminish and the difference between citizen and outlaw becomes inconstant and unclear. The more we know about the aging body—and the aging immune system—the more it resembles an aging civilization.

BETWEEN CELLS

Most of us have the impression that cells are crammed in, squeezed elbow to elbow, with no space between them. Your cells are indeed often tightly packed, but the space that remains is another critical part of aging. This border zone, the matrix between cells, is packed with proteins and a stew of molecules with many jobs and functions that are often less understood than those of the cells that surround them. These molecules are the nails and rafters that hold cells together and support much of the structure they rely on. These proteins and other molecules are also pools that your cells recycle in a slow, continuous process over the years.

As cells age, they alter the way they interact with their fellow cells, and with the proteins and other molecules inhabiting the borders between them. As your cells age, they break down more of their surrounding matrix but are slower, or unable, to replace it. Aging cells not only are unable to recycle and replace the matrix between them, but they put out inflammatory signals, inciting the immune system to do further damage.

The alteration is subtle, but universal: Anywhere cells approach the end of their clocks the matrix shows changes, and the neighboring cells are distressed and altered. Aging is not a local phenomenon. The aging of one cell is the problem of the entire neighborhood and, ultimately, of distant but fellow cells.

Y O U R   B O D Y

I am ready to meet my maker, but whether my maker is prepared for the great ordeal of meeting me is another matter.

—WINSTON CHURCHILL

Aging is not local, but universal. Telomeres shorten; bodies age. It is not only the individual cell that ages, but groups of cells. And it's not even mere groups of cells that age, but the entire body. Each cell differs. Some have not divided since we first opened our eyes; some are dividing hourly. Some have long telomeres, some short ones, some almost none at all. Some cells live and prosper and some die, but throughout our lives, everywhere in our bodies, all of our cells depend on one another. You are not a mere collection of cells, but an arrangement—intricate and miraculous—of hundreds of trillions of cells in a design that will never be duplicated and that never remains the same.

Our bodies age for a thousand reasons, but most of our aging can be traced back to the clocks that lie in each of our cells, the ninety-two separately ticking clocks. Some of our cells age because they run out of time, others because their neighbors do. Some of our systems are old because their cells are old, others because of other systems that are old. These bystanders that undergo aging indirectly, do so not in simple, uniform fashion; rather they trip over the debris of other aging cells and systems, falling into haphazard but certain disaster. They crack, weaken, and rust, whether because of their own slowing clocks or because of clocks elsewhere that have run out of time. The cascade of damage is so universal and thorough that—until now—it has eluded explanation, and yet left us certain of its inevitability.

Our *actual* life span is determined not only by our telomeres, but also by all the genes that lie between those telomeres. If you die at birth, the fault was in your genes, not your telomeres. The older you get, the more your life span is determined by your telomeres. Our *maximum* life span is determined by *our telomeres*. It is the longest time that each of us would live if our genes and our environment didn't otherwise kill us.

As we have become better and better at living longer, the telomeres have finally come to decide our fate. They decide not only when we will die, but what diseases we will suffer from and finally succumb to now that we live long enough for them to matter. They represent the clocks that undermine the efforts of our genes to protect us from the world. The telomeres are not alone in this undermining, however. If we were to reverse their shortening, we would expose ourselves to a multitude of yet unknown weaknesses that our gene libraries have in store for us, weaknesses that have never been a problem when death came as early as it does now.

Many of these genetic weaknesses are not yet evident because our telomeres are currently the final hurdle that none of us overcomes. We pass obstacle after obstacle on our way through life, only to find our feet slipping out from beneath us as our clocks run down. Resetting our clocks will not allow us to live forever; it will only put us back in the obstacle course, subject to the same problems that all living things must face, even under the best of circumstances.

The obstacle course is complex. Not only must each cell achieve its own delicate balance, but so must groups of cells and the entire body. A cell must do more than just survive; it must coordinate its survival with hundreds of trillions of other cells. Any mistake, if large enough, can destroy this balance.

That destruction is exactly what occurs in aging. The balance is destroyed progressively as more and more cells, losing their abilities, drag down otherwise healthy cells. Each failing cell increases the risk of its neighbor's failure. Each failing organ increases the risk of failure elsewhere. Each failure increases the risk of our death.

Aging is a universal process. It affects all cells, all systems, all organs.

It increases the threat posed by every bad gene we carry and it decreases the protective value of our every good gene. It increases our risks of dying from almost every disease.

Death is almost always due to disease, and that becomes increasingly likely as we grow older. Rarely is death a purely entropic affair; but if we are hit by a car at sufficient speed, our age, our telomeres, our homeostatic defenses are all irrelevant. On a less catastrophic and more common level, our telomeres contribute strongly to our chances of living out the day.

In some cases, however, the telomeres are outvoted substantially. Some genes are so poor that no one survives long enough for telomeres to make a difference. Children with severe immune deficiency don't die because they have no telomeres, but because they have no immune system. Any major genetic problem may render your telomeres moot. Even minor problems are sometimes only peripherally related to telomeres. As we age, we lose our teeth. The timing may be influenced by our telomeres, but no matter how long our telomeres, we still receive only two sets of teeth. Reextending our telomeres is no substitute for brushing, good diet, and dental care.

Telomeres don't make new teeth and telomeres don't make new genes, but they do influence how our genes play out and, more important, how long we might have to let them work. The telomeres express themselves not in whether we have good genes or bad, but in whether they are allowed to function normally as we age. They do not determine whether or not we live, but whether or not we age. Aging is caused by aging cells and aging cells by aging telomeres.

CHAPTER 6

TURNING BACK THE CLOCK

A NEW TIME

There is a plant that grows under water, it has a prickle like a thorn, like a rose; it will wound your hands, but if you succeed in taking it, then your hands will hold that which restores his lost youth to a man.

—*THE EPIC OF GILGAMESH*

FOR MOST OF us, intellectual theories of aging are irrelevant. Few of us actually care exactly how a disease works or whether people can agree on the mechanism of aging. And concerning the therapies for reversing aging, most of us are simply interested in their effectiveness. We are less concerned with what causes cancer than with whether it can be cured. We want to know what will work.

By its very nature, any attempt to increase the human life span by altering the telomere will involve an alteration of chromosomes and, roughly speaking, genes. There are several types of gene therapy, each with its own ethical implications.[1] For example, does the therapy aim at the somatic or germ cells? Does it aim to correct a genetic disease, or is it only a cosmetic concern?

The somatic-versus-germ-cell debate is essential because it pinpoints the distinction between whether you would be affecting only yourself (somatic cells) or future generations (germ cells). Gene alterations in somatic cells raises fewer, or at least different, objections than does alteration of your germ cells. After all, these future generations that are affected by changes in germ cells are not consulted in your decision.

There is also the muddy distinction between alteration for the purpose of curing or preventing disease and for purely cosmetic purposes, which two rationales make up the poles of a moral spectrum. Cancer is a disease; preventing and curing it is good. Eye color and hair color are not diseases; but cosmetic characteristics; Changing, not "curing," them is neither good nor bad. To do so raises three issues: cost, risk, and "sanctity." With respect to cost, to use limited resources to effect cosmetic changes at the expense of changes that could prevent and cure diseases, is clearly unethical. Concerning medical risk, if the risk of altering your genes is high, then we must weigh it against the value of the desired results. High risk may be ethically acceptable in treating an otherwise fatal cancer, but not when only a cosmetic change is made. The issue of the "sanctity" of our genes is the most intangible and problematic one we must face in dealing with the prospect of gene alteration. That sanctity is assumed but is rarely mentioned in discussions of this issue. Most of us feel that any genetic alteration must be for a reason sufficiently important that it justifies not only the cost and the risk involved, but also the effrontery of changing the blueprints of life. For example, Nelson Wivel, director of the Office of Recombinant DNA Activities at the National Institutes of Health, and LeRoy Walters, a professor of ethics at Georgetown University, wrote an article on the ethics of genetic manipulation in *Science* magazine, in which they worried that "genetic modification ... could be directed toward healthy people who have no evidence of genetic deficiency diseases."[2] The assumption is that the genes should be left alone unless there is a deficiency disease.

One problem with this assumption is that "deficiency" and "disease" are both slippery terms. Deficiency of immune response is a disease, whereas a generalized deficiency of melanin among Caucasians is probably not. But what about a deficiency of neural connections in the brain? How low does one's IQ have to be to qualify as a deficiency? What about height? How low must your growth hormone level—or any other factor—be to qualify as a genetic deficiency disease?

What about menopause? It is universal, natural, and normal among women who live long enough. It seems clear that it is not a disease, yet the medical "complications" linked to it make us think of it as a disease. Menopause increases the risk of osteoporosis and, consequently, of fractures. Fractured bones hurt and may require surgery, and the risk of death climbs from both the fracture and the surgery. Menopause also increases the risk of other potentially fatal diseases, such as coronary artery disease, which leads to cardiac death. Most women tolerate the hot flashes and mucosal changes of menopause, while the onset of cardiac risk is more gradual and only distantly attributed to menopause. However, many women and physicians are eager to, at least partially, reverse menopause and its attendant increase in morbidity and mortality.

The question of whether menopause is a disease is debated. Menopause is universal, natural, unavoidable, and genetic, and in this sense is not a disease. But it is also often uncomfortable, occasionally dangerous, rarely fatal, and can be altered, and in this other sense, it is a disease, one that many already seek treatment for. So how should we define it, by our words or by our actions? We might argue that it is a disease because people treat it like one; they dislike it and they try to change it.

In a similar sense, we can ask if aging is a disease. We have always believed that aging is not a disease. It is universal, natural, unavoidable, and genetic. Although many biologists argue aggressively against defining aging as a disease, it is easy to see how we could think of it as one. Suffering from it, watching our parents slowly succumb to it or our spouse reap its pain and complications, make us reconsider the superficial merits of a narrow definition. The question of whether aging is a disease is not genetic, biological, or even medical; it is human.

The important question, after all, is, given an opportunity to alter aging's course, do people treat it like a disease? Do they complain about it and try to avoid it? Do they try to treat it and want to prevent or reverse it? They certainly do.

Not universally, not always, not without second thoughts, but generally, people act as though aging were a disease. By the force of their actions, they define it as the final, underlying, universal disease. It is not infectious, or accidental, or the result of a genetic error. To the contrary, genes enforce it with vengeance and vigor. It is a natural and a normal part of our biology. But it is not easy and it is not, to most people, desirable. Although aging does not fit the biologist's definition of a disease, it becomes defined as one by our emotions and actions.

REVERSAL

We are here to add what we can to, not get what we can from, life.

—WILLIAM OSLER

Aging is an ascending disorder—it slowly takes apart the order that is life. It starts at the telomere and culminates in your wholesale disorder and death. At what level then do we treat aging? We could start at the grossest level, replacing your heart, using dialysis instead of young kidneys, and adding titanium and plastic where your bone once grew and supported you. These approaches are losing battles, which would be quickly overcome and evaded by a body whose functions are evaporating with age. In addition, they are expensive, inefficient, and insufficient.

We could go deeper into your organism and find ways to more efficiently repair your DNA damage, restore function to your leaky membranes, and replace your old mitochondria. This would still not strike deeply enough. At yet deeper levels, we might remove your free radicals, reverse isomerization of your molecules, and build better defenses against high-energy photons. But none of these approaches would be able to overcome the universal and ubiquitous ticking of our clocks.

The telomere is only place where all the mechanisms of aging come together, and it is here where we can most efficiently prevent or reverse the myriad dysfunctions that express themselves as aging. It is here that we can reverse aging.

The two major approaches to adjusting the telomeric clock are to reset it and stop it. Both have been accomplished in cells. Researchers at the University of Texas Southwest Medical Center can reset the telomeric clocks in fibroblasts. These techniques allow us to reset or even stop their telomeric clocks, and continue to grow them indefinitely. Before considering how this could be done in your entire body, it is important to examine what can be done to individual cells.

The telomere shortens because every time the cell divides, it fails to copy the tips of its chromosomes. Chromosome copying starts at a primer, which often binds downstream from the actual end of the telomere. When it comes off, the underlying telomere never gets copied, which causes it to shorten. What if we locked a permanent primer on the end of each telomere so that copying would always start at this "lock" and always copy the full telomere (including the lock itself)? Adenoviruses and pox viruses do this already. The result would be that the telomere wouldn't shorten. The clock, still fully wound up, would be permanently stopped.

Researchers at the University of Texas have already done this to human cells in culture, by building "caps" out of the same nucleic acids that make up the chromosome.[3] These cells no longer have a Hayflick limit. They no longer age. On the other hand, they don't get any younger, either. A young cell stays permanently young, an old cell stays permanently old. Can't we do better than just stopping the clock? Can't we reset it?

All we need to do is increase the length of the telomere, which would reset gene expression, allow the cell to cycle normally, and leave a younger cell. And when it ran down again, at the same pace it did the first time, we could rewind it again. We could even try locking it in place after we rewind it. That would give us a cell that had been rewound and stayed that way.

The simplest approach to relengthening, or "rewinding," the telomeres in cell cultures is to add telomerase, which makes the cell act exactly as it did when it was first cultured: It divides normally and produces protein normally. If the cell had a life span of fifty divisions and we reset its clock when it has only five left, it would start all over again with another fifty divisions. And the second time around, it wouldn't age any faster than it did the first. The clock would have been completely reset.

Telomerase is not naturally found in most human cells, although the gene for it is present in every cell.[4] Even though researchers at Cold Spring Harbor and at the Geron Corporation are close to uncovering the complete human telomerase structure, currently they still isolate it from the few organisms that manufacture telomerase in large enough quantities, such as tetrahymena. While it is easy enough to put telomerase into cells in a culture dish, introducing it into normal cells in an entire body is another matter. Telomerase is fragile and readily destroyed by the normal enzymes in your blood. Its half-life in your bloodstream is so short that it won't work when we simply inject telomerase into your blood; it has barely arrived at your cells before it is gone, and it never reaches your chromosomes at all.

While normal telomerase administered by vein won't reset our trillions of cellular clocks, there are three other ways of resetting the telomere: We could administer either a telomerase analog, or a gene that would express telomerase, or an inducer that would unlock your own telomerase gene. A telomerase analog would be an artificial telomerase that was tougher and more durable than normal telomerase. This is commonly done with antibiotics, steroids, and other useful molecules by making small chemical changes in the original molecule— adding fluorine or a methyl group, for example. Molecules of "synthetic telomerase" that aren't broken down by your body for hours or days might effectively lengthen your telomeres, evade destruction, and extend the lives of your cells. The telomerase analog could be given by injection and would last long enough to enter your cells and reset their telomeres before finally being broken down. A single course of treatment would lengthen your telomeres and start reversing the effects of aging on your body. The work on this approach has barely begun: Researchers only published the structure of the RNA portion (the protein portion is still unknown) of human telomerase in 1995.[5] We still need to be able to produce human telomerase in the laboratory before we can alter it to create a more durable molecule and an effective treatment. What we could do, even now, is to administer telomerase to particular cells that show aging problems, for example, the endothelial cells of your blood vessels. We could insert a "double balloon catheter" into the vessels, temporarily interrupt blood flow, flush the small portion of the vessel between the two obstructing balloons with telomerase, then remove the catheter. That would reset the telomeres of the endothelial cells in that part of the blood vessel. We could cure vascular disease, and so prevent heart disease.

The second approach is to construct genes that manufacture telomerase in normal somatic cells. Since your telomerase genes are normally repressed and therefore won't make telomerase, we could give your cells new genes that would. This approach would avoid having to force the telomerase through the gauntlet of the bloodstream and into the hundreds of trillions of cells in the body. Using the new genes, each cell would make its own telomerase and extend its own life span. There are numerous problems with this approach, mainly deriving from the fact that we currently know only part of the sequences of human telomerase. How can we build genes for the entire enzyme, when we don't know the whole sequence yet? Once we have learned the full DNA sequences, we need to build an artificial gene that produces telomerase. We need to insert the sequences into a viral carrier or a liposome,[6] inject it into the body, have it infect every one of your 100 trillion cells, and express telomerase reliably.[7]

We should not be optimistic about the insertion of a telomerase gene. We have managed to insert viral genes into small numbers of cells, but not by injecting the virus into the bloodstream or targeting every cell in the entire body. Currently, the technique for using viral carriers to cure genetic illnesses involves taking cells out of the body, infecting them with a virus that carries the necessary gene, then reinserting the altered cells. Alternatively, we sometimes administer the virus to small areas of tissue, such as the lung (by inhalation).

Research in this field is progressing fast enough that we are likely to know the entire sequences, including the protein portion, for human telomerase within the next two years. Building the genes to code for it is relatively easy, even now. Finding a workable carrier is still slightly difficult, but within five years we will probably be using this approach on aging tissue, such as coronary arteries. Just as with telomerase, we could use a double balloon catheter to deliver the virus to damaged arteries, reset their telomeres, and reverse the damage to the vessel walls.

A final problem remains with this second approach, however. Even if the viral carrier is able to deliver the gene to every cell, how much telomerase will the cell produce? Will the new gene manufacture enough, or perhaps too much, telomerase? It is not enough to place functioning telomerase genes in each cell; we must control how much telomerase they produce. Otherwise the cell might build enormous telomeres. What if the cell can't divide or can't access its genes normally because the superlong telomere is in the way? What about the increased risk of cancer if telomeres are too long? Not only do we need to deliver the telomerase gene to each cell, but we need to build in gene regulation along with it. We need to be able to express telomerase in each cell, but we also need to control it.

The third approach, perhaps the best, would be to induce your own genes to produce telomerase. After all, every one of your somatic cells already *has* telomerase genes. While either of the first two approaches may be feasible, and might even be the one we settle on in the decades to come, the last approach is the most elegant. Why not simply "turn on" the genes that are already there?

Researchers are currently working on all three approaches. The first approach—creating an artificial telomerase—requires that we complete our search for the human telomerase sequence; the second—creating and inserting a new gene—requires that we learn more about both the sequence and viral carriers; whereas the third—"turning on" our own genes—requires only dogged work and luck. In the third approach, researchers are screening hundreds of thousands of compounds to find one that activates the telomerase gene. That is exactly the same approach which has already resulted in one of the two families of telomerase inhibitors to treat cancer. The dose of the drug, how effective it is, and how fast it breaks down would determine how much telomerase you make and, indirectly, how much your telomeres lengthen.

One potential problem may actually be a help. The cell actively suppresses telomerase genes.[8] That may work to our advantage, by enhancing our ability to control them. When we administer a telomerase inducer, the cell will produce telomerase, but when we stop administering the inducer, the production will be self-limiting, as though it had braked itself and came to rest without any further treatment on our part.

Our best bet for a drug to extend our health spans would be a telomerase inducer. Active research programs for such a drug are being conducted at the University of Texas Southwestern University Medical Center and at Cold Spring Harbor Laboratory, as well as through agreements with other biotechnology and pharmaceutical firms. Most large pharmaceutical firms have "drug libraries" containing hundreds of thousands of drugs—and their formulas—that might have therapeutic uses, but usually don't. Each drug is identified chemically, but its potential uses remain unknown until they can be screened for a particular therapeutic effect. Researchers are screening such libraries for both telomerase inhibition—for cancer therapy—and telomerase induction—for aging and age-related disease. The screening is laborious, but straightforward, and has already resulted in several telomerase inhibitors. The search for telomerase inducers is quite likely to be equally successful within the next year or so.

There is yet another approach worth mentioning. Why not simply disconnect the clock, turning off its consequences? Could we not find some inhibitor of the DDBP proteins that detect the end of the telomere? Why not end-run the timing mechanism? Such an approach is unworkable because nature doesn't allow cells to survive without telomeres. Even cancer cells do not evade the clock mechanism; they become immortal by resetting their clocks, by relengthening their telomeres. Those that don't, die. All malignant cells express telomerase to survive.[9]

Resetting the telomere is the only mechanism that nature uses to let these cells survive beyond their normal number of divisions. In some living things, we find cells that have no clocks. In other forms of life, we find cells with clocks that don't run down. Nowhere does any form of life simply let the clock run down and then survive it. If the entire telomere structure is eaten away and the genes themselves begin to disappear, the cell dies. If we want to reverse aging, we might best follow nature's example and try resetting them.

TREATING DISEASE

The first diseases treated with telomere alteration will probably be progeria, vessel disease, and cancer. Why? In the case of progeria, there are three reasons: The cause of the disease is short telomeres, everyone agrees that it *is* a disease, and there is no other form of treatment. Although the exact mechanisms of some aging-related diseases—Alzheimer's dementia, for instance—are unclear, in the case of progeria the outcome appears to be direct: short telomeres, short lives.

In addition, everyone agrees that progeria, vessel disease, and cancer are diseases and therefore need treatment, whereas some will initially argue against treating aging on the grounds that it isn't a disease. Finally, progeria, unlike cancer or vessel disease, has *no* current treatment; telomerase induction promises to change that.

The first progeric child will be treated with a telomerase inducer within the next ten years. The child will probably be admitted to a research hospital—perhaps under the care of Dr. Ted Brown in New York, currently the world's leading clinician for progeria—where he or she will be given a series of tests—blood, EKG, X rays, pulmonary function, urine, and so forth—to establish baseline function prior to treatment. The first dose of a telomerase inducer will be placed into a normal, unremarkable IV bag and given to the child over a few hours. The results will be undramatic for a number of days at least. When they occur, the first changes will be modest but tangible: The child's energy level will increase, the appetite will improve, there will be fewer aches and pains. The child will be discharged, returning periodically once a week to be rechecked. More marked improvement will be noticed within a handful of weeks as the skin, circulation, kidneys, and other organs very gradually improve. As months pass, there will be improvement in cardiac function and arthritic joints. As the first year passes, the child's health will begin to approach normal. But long before the year is out, other progeric children will begin treatment and the implications for treating normal aging with telomerase inducers will be inevitable.

Treating vessel disease with a telomerase inducer will be tried first in animals—animals don't get progeria, but some of them do acquire vessel disease—within the next two years or so, followed soon thereafter by trials on humans. Initially, a catheter will be placed directly in the diseased vessel, rather than administering the drug systemically through a routine intravenous line. "Clot busting" agents, such as streptokinase, were initially used the same way, being administered by a catheter in the coronary arteries and only later becoming accepted for use through normal IV lines. Once we understand the efficacy and safety of telomerase therapy, we will begin to try it on other diseases related to aging cells. The result will be a flood of clinical uses.

The work on telomerase inhibitors is more advanced than the work on inducers; cancer therapy will precede therapy for aging. Two families of telomerase inhibitors are currently undergoing trials in animals. The first human trials cannot be far off: The best estimates from those working with these compounds is before 2000.[10] A reasonable estimate is that if the rate of development continues, we will have a clinically available cure for most cancers by the year 2005 or soon thereafter. A cancer patient will be diagnosed one day, begin treatment the next, and expect clinical results within a matter of weeks. Telomerase inhibitors should not affect normal cells; there should be few, if any, side effects. We will no longer have vomiting, lost hair, and immune suppression as the routine costs of cancer therapy. Therapy will probably consist of several intravenous treatments, daily or perhaps once a week, over a few weeks until the cancer is gone. In some cases, additional therapy may be needed: Single tumors might be easily removed surgically as they are now; telomerase inhibitors might work better or faster if accompanied by other drugs, similar to those we use now.

But will cancer get worse when we treat aging with a telomerase inducer? Premalignant cells would be given a slightly freer rein by being allowed a few more cell divisions to try to become fully malignant. However, therapeutic use of telomerase doesn't make premalignant cells immortal and it doesn't make them into cancer cells. Malignant cells would likewise be given a few more cell divisions, even though they already have endless ones; their own expression of telomerase already allows them a precarious but continuous immortality. Telomerase therapy adds nothing that they don't already have.

Treating aging with telomerase inducers would slightly increase our chances of acquiring cancer; but we would also treat ourselves with a telomerase inhibitor to kill cancers before commencing telomerase therapy. And we would be ready to kill cancer cells safely and efficiently if they occurred later as well. Telomerase inhibitors shut down telomerase production in cancer cells, pushing forward their clocks until they die. This has already been done in the laboratory in cancerous HeLa cells by forcing them to make their own telomerase inhibitor— a so-called "antisense RNA" that blocks the action of normal telomerase.[11] Once treated, cancer cells age themselves to death with no cost to normal cells, which don't normally express telomerase anyway. Not only will cancer soon be curable, but we will have little to fear from cancer when we reverse aging in your normal cells.

Progeria and cancer are not the only diseases affected by the telomere, however. We can do several things that were previously impossible. One major obstacle to growing organs—human skin, for instance—was the Hayflick limit: Cells could only be induced to grow for a limited number of divisions before they died. We will soon be able to overcome that limit and grow—"*ex vivo*," out of the body—any tissue that we can make divide and are capable of supporting, in any amount we need to. We will be able to provide human skin for transplanting onto burn victims. Diabetics may have new pancreatic cells, hepatitis victims new livers; others might someday have new hearts, new lungs, and new blood vessels. AIDS patients might have new white blood stem cells, others new red blood stem cells; the possibilities are hypothetical and still unexplored, but they are also enormous.

YOU

Imagine that you are seventy, with the typical blood vessels and organs of someone that old. You are active and healthy, but the years have made changes. How long will it take to reverse them? Initially, you might guess that it would take as long as it did to create the damage. After all, your telomeres required time to erode; it took different cells varying amounts of time to fall prey to aging. But resetting your telomeres will be a more uniform process; they might all be reset within days of treatment. Although the resetting of the clocks could be fairly uniform and rapid, and although the time it would require could be independent of how long it took you and your cells to age, that still doesn't tell us how long it would be before we saw any change in you. Cells are one thing, you are another.

In your blood vessels, a single endothelial cell, previously unable to divide and protect your vessel wall, would now almost immediately, perhaps within hours of treatment, be capable of division again. It would then divide and provide better coverage of the inner wall. But how soon would the cholesterol deposits, macrophage cells, and other signs of inflammation recede, leaving the vessel open and smooth? Predicting that is a chancy affair, but most likely it would take sometime between weeks and years. Our only information on this matter comes from the results of drastic and thorough changes in people's diets, for example, as occurred during the World War II occupation of the Netherlands. Whether it is accomplished medically or by famine, the vessels slowly improve and the risk of heart disease falls, but the improvement takes time; usually many months. The changes occur faster with strict starvation than they do with partial dietary changes, but the result is the same: Cholesterol levels fall and so do deaths due to vessel disease.

Telomere therapy affecting other body systems will probably take similar amounts of time. Telomeres might be extended almost immediately, but clinical changes will take more time. As we will see in the next chapter, some clinical improvements will never occur. We cannot expect to regain brain cells that have died, but we can expect to stop losing them to disease caused by aging cells.

Another positive aspect of telomere therapy is a lack of "payback." We will not have to worry about reaching the age of 150 and then suddenly aging in a single day or year. Aging, whether it is "the first time" or after telomere therapy, works slowly. It takes time because your cells divide over a period of decades as they are needed. Telomere therapy doesn't change the *speed* of cellular aging; it just changes the number of years it will take your body to grow old. Even in progeric children, where aging appears accelerated, the pace of the underlying process is the same as it is in normal ones, but their cells *start out* old. They look old in only a few years because all their telomeres are already shorter at birth—so aging appears abbreviated.

In fact, if telomere therapy makes your telomeres long enough, it will take even longer than it normally would before your body acts aged. Your cells will divide just as fast, your telomeres will shorten just as fast, but if your clocks are wound further than they are in the normal young adult, it will take longer to become old.

Whether it takes decades or a century, repeat treatment will be necessary unless we lock the telomeres in place, which might further increase the risk of cancer. The conservative approach, at least initially, will probably be simply to reextend the telomere periodically. Considering how long it currently takes your body to mature and how long it takes to age, you might reasonably expect to need retreatment every few decades.

The treatments will likely work as they do in the following scenario:

Despite the unknowns, at age seventy you decide to try your first treatment. You have moderate arthritis. Stairs are impossible; getting out of bed in the morning is a chore. Your heart isn't what it once was: You use nitroglycerin pills about once a week for an annoying chest pressure that you feel when you overdo it; you tire easily and can't catch your breath just walking to the bus stop, and usually have to rest a few times to make it. You fell while boarding the bus last month and had to have stitches in your arm; it still hasn't healed. Even with all this, you count yourself lucky compared with many of your friends.

Still, you'd like more from life than shortness of breath, arthritis, and chest pain, so you make an appointment. The first day you have a few blood tests and an examination. The second day, you are given a pill; the nurse checks your blood pressure, and watches you for half an hour before sending you home. But before you get home, the pill has already dissolved and the active ingredient—a telomerase inducer—has already started into your bloodstream. Within an hour, some of your cells have begun to express telomerase. By nightfall, your cells are resetting their own telomeres. A week later, you're back. You haven't noticed any changes. Your blood pressure is the same, as are your other tests. The doctor points out that the scrape on your arm has finally healed beautifully, and you notice that your liver spots are fading a bit and your skin is firmer and healthier. A month passes before your next visit and you haven't had any chest pressure for a week. Your arthritis didn't bother you as much during the past two or three days, but the weather has been warmer. After the exam is over, you think about stopping at the library on the way home; you haven't had the energy to go there for a few years, but you've been eating better this week now that your appetite is better. Then you change your mind about the library and decide to go out to lunch.

Six months have passed and you have only seen your doctor once in that time. You stopped by to thank him after you played tennis for the first time in ten years. You and a friend have been traveling again. Even when you're back home, there are so many other things to do that you keep putting it off. Maybe next month, if the bicycle you ordered comes, you might ride over and see what the doctor thinks of you. Maybe, if you can fit it in between tennis games.

PREVENTION

When I was one, I had just begun. When I was two, I was
*   nearly new.*
When I was three, I was hardly me. When I was four, I was
*   not much more.*
When I was five, I was just alive. But now I am six, I'm as
*   clever as clever.*
So I think I'll be six now for ever and ever.

—A. A. MILNE, NOW WE ARE SIX

Reversing aging is more difficult than preventing it. It is easier to prevent damage from occurring than it is to repair that which has already happened. Clearly, if we wait too long, the therapy will not be as effective as it might have been. But is there a lower age limit to its use as well?

If we treat children, there is little advantage, except in progeric children, and we should be concerned that we might interfere with their maturation. But maturation isn't determined by telomeres. In progeric children, for example, maturation progresses in a normal order, even though the telomeres are short. Longer telomeres shouldn't change the order and pace of maturation either.

While telomere therapy will bring us back to the body of a fully developed young adult, it will not prevent maturation or return an adult to a child's body. The length of the telomere does not determine maturation, but aging. By lengthening the telomeres, the body will become that of a young adult; however, some functions will be more like those of a child. For instance, adult healing is notoriously slower and less complete than healing in children. Infants have occasionally regrown entire fingers; adults never do. After telomere therapy, we might expect to regain the modest degree of regenerative ability seen in the average, normal child.[12] But even this possibility could depend on cells that may be lost if we wait too long before having telomere therapy.

Telomere therapy will probably offer little advantage to the child, some to the young adult, and considerable advantage to the older person. The best range of ages for such therapy, if we want to prevent aging and age-related disease, will be between sixteen and forty. Sixteen is probably a bit too early to gain any benefit and forty a bit too late to avoid the risk of *some* irreversible changes. Anyone older will benefit enormously, but not as much as they might have, had they prevented aging in the first place, rather than reversing *almost* all of it. The optimal age depends very much on each person's own pattern of aging. A progeric child will need to be treated as soon as possible, perhaps at age two. Some adults, whose genes are allowing them to age more slowly than their peers, may decide to delay treatment until they see how others do. They will be playing a dangerous game, however, which they will lose if their cells fail them unexpectedly. The optimal use of telomere therapy is not to reverse aging, but to prevent it.

SAVING YOUR OWN LIFE

Whosoever enjoys not this life, I count him but an apparition . . . the way to be immortal is to die daily.

—THOMAS BROWNE

Telomere alteration will dramatically affect your health and your life span, but it is not a panacea. It won't make you invulnerable to automobile accidents or assaults, it won't guarantee that you will not die of any disease you might otherwise acquire, and it won't make your genes any better than they are now.

Because telomere therapy lowers your chances of a heart attack, that doesn't mean you won't have one. It doesn't necessarily make it safer to eat foods high in cholesterol; it just makes a heart attack less likely. There will still be every bit as much reason to exercise, to avoid saturated fats, to stop smoking, and to pursue any other course of action that you are now to maintain your health.

Consider the situation of a tree. It could fall down because of a heavy wind blowing it over, or because of an ax chopping its trunk, or because of a saw cutting through it. If all of these things happened simultaneously, the tree would fall quickly. But any one of them could take it down eventually. If you were the tree, the wind would be aging, the ax high cholesterol, and the saw high blood pressure. If the wind was strong, it wouldn't take the ax or the saw long to weaken the tree enough to make it fall. However, if the wind stopped, the tree would still fall, but the cut would have to go deeper before the tree failed. The same is true with aging. Even if we stop the wind that buffets and tears at the tree, if we continue to chop away (with enough cholesterol) or saw at it (with a high enough blood pressure), sooner or later our arteries will fail, our heart will die, and so will we. A still wind doesn't protect your body from axes, saws, or from behaving foolishly. And cholesterol and high blood pressure are only two of a thousand enemies, including infection, trauma, cancer, and a host of others.

Even with telomere therapy, you still have the same genes you always had. Some have your course set for cancer, some for heart disease, and some for diseases you wouldn't have lived long enough to fall prey to had you not had telomere therapy.

To extend your life and maintain your health, you not only need to extend your telomeres, but eat a high-fiber and low-fat diet rich in fruits and vegetables,[13] exercise, avoid stress, and take every opportunity to avoid, detect, and treat diseases that you might contract someday. You should do exactly the same things you would do even without telomere therapy.

It is as though entropy were an escalator going down, and homeostasis were you, walking up. Maintaining a balance, you stay in one place until the slowing of your clock forces you to stop walking and the escalator carries you down. Even when we rewind the clock, however, there is no percentage in consciously turning around and walking *down* the escalator, which you do when you have an unhealthy diet, encourage disease, and court disaster.

Currently, without changing your telomeres at all, there are thousands of positive suggestions for living longer. If slight increases in dietary vitamin E and C really lower your risk of arterial disease—they probably do, but there are more cautious voices[14]—they will continue to do so following telomere therapy. If Retin-A is effective against wrinkles, it still will be; if meditation lowers your stress and makes you healthier, it too still will be; if some therapy, promoted for delaying aging, is actively dangerous, it will still be, even if your telomeres are reset and locked in place.

The aging process can be influenced at any number of levels, but the results depend on where we intervene. If we alter the clock, we can reset the entire process, by and large. If we only change the turn-over rates for your proteins, then we only change those things that are affected by that turnover rate. If we only decrease free radicals, we will alter only the part of aging affected by free radicals. If vitamins E and C lower the damage caused by free radicals, that will affect part of the aging process, but not all of it; it won't cure aging, but it could have beneficial effects.

But what if a particular vitamin supplement also has a few, minimal detrimental effects? What if it actually causes damage, but the effect is usually lost amid its overwhelmingly good effects on aging? If we reset your aging clock and free radical damage was minimized, so that we perhaps wouldn't *need* as much of these vitamins, why should we take a vitamin supplement? Given enough time—now that you live another few hundred years—the side effects of high doses might become noticeable and even fatal. Perhaps the slight detrimental effects of vitamin C on kidney function—stone formation, for example—became overwhelming after taking large doses regularly for fifty years. Retinoids might increase your risk of kidney disease; vitamin C and beta carotene might damage the heart and vitamin E increase your risk of stroke.[15] These effects would become the only important ones remaining if vessel disease were effectively prevented by telomere therapy, allowing us no rationale for tolerating the unopposed, potential detrimental effects of vitamin supplements.

The same concerns apply to DHEA, melatonin, growth hormone, gerovital, conjugated water, procaine, and any other purported aging therapy. They might be beneficial in the short run (a few decades), but disastrous in the long run (a few centuries). We are likely to find new diseases and problems when we extend the human life span, but currently there is no way to predict them.

If telomere therapy does extend our life spans as we expect it will, it becomes even more important that you care for your body wisely. A car leased for six months needs the oil changed, but if it has to last ten years, every nick and rust spot, loose bolt, drop of dirty oil, and few degrees of wheel alignment will affect how well it works. In 1900, life expectancy was 25 years and no one cared about high cholesterol. Knowing you could live to be 250, you will recognize the importance of taking care of your arteries and other organs from the beginning. They will determine your life span; they will become your weakest links.

To extend your life and stay healthy as long as possible, you will have to do not only everything that makes sense now, but more. As we reset our clocks to extend our life spans, exercise, a good diet, stress avoidance, all the fads and fancies that we so ardently—often foolishly—believe, become even smarter, or stupider. How far you extend your life span will depend on the care you give your body and also on how well you sort fact from fad.

CAN WE DO IT?

The period of rapid increase in human life expectation . . . has ended. . . . An enormous effect might occur if we could reduce to the level of young cells, the susceptibility of old cells to . . . diseases.

—LEONARD HAYFLICK, *HOW AND WHY WE AGE*

Your life span can be extended by several hundred years. The technical hurdles appear enormous, but so were the ones involved in going to the moon, building a computer, or sequencing a human gene. These obstacles too will be overcome sometime within the next decade.

Consider what stands in our way. We must figure out how to lengthen the telomeres (all ninety-two of them) in each of your cells (all 100 trillion of them). "All" we need to do is to add a few thousand DNA bases to each of roughly 10 quadrillion molecules in your body. How can we do this? The methods are few, but they are promising.

Earlier in this chapter, we discussed the methods we could use to reset the telomere and reverse aging. Let's look more closely at the most likely method. Remember the library analogy: Somewhere in one of the chromosomal books in each of the genetic libraries in every cell in your body, there are a few sentences that tell how to make telomerase.[16] We know they are there; although almost none of your somatic cells make telomerase, those that transform into a cancer always do. The sentence, or blueprint, for producing telomerase is in every one of your cells to be put to use. We need to find the key, the same type that unlocks telomerase in germ cells.

We don't have to treat 10 quadrillion telomeres; we have to treat perhaps 100 trillion cells, and each cell can treat its own 92 telomeres. Is this feasible? In the simplest terms, most chemicals that you ingest penetrate everywhere; how fast they penetrate and their final concentration depends on whether the chemical dissolves better in water or in fat, how acidic it is, how large it is, and its exact shape. But given enough time and a high enough dose, any chemical will go anywhere we want it to go. The important questions now are not about penetration but whether the drug will work and whether we can afford such a drug.

Telomere therapy will be too expensive to be fair and too inexpensive to be believable. Most of us in the developed world would consider an extended health span as a bargain at any price. We would most likely mortgage our homes and extend our debt to buy a healthier, longer life. But even in the United States, Europe, Japan, and Australia, there are limits to what we can afford. If the price of a treatment were half the average income, it would still be more than many could afford. In the poorer countries of the world, many cannot afford tetanus vaccine, let alone telomere therapy. No matter what the price, some will find it impossible, whereas almost all will find it a bargain. The price is likely to be reasonable. The major costs will involve the original research itself and the clinical trials; the costs of production and distribution will be far less. The current research costs are modest by comparison with most developments in pharmaceuticals and in genetic therapy. In terms of the latter, we need the telomere lengthened or the telomere gene turned on, not inserted into your genes. All of these factors will determine the range of the drug price, which, for a single treatment of telomerase induction, is likely to be between $50 and $1,000.[17]

Another reason telomere therapy will be inexpensive is the potentially vast market. Some won't want it, some will die of other diseases while too young to need it, but the market will still be large. The wider the market, the lower the per capita costs. A full treatment of most current drugs is typically less than $100. Many of these are cheap because their research costs have been paid off long ago. The larger the market for any drug, the sooner the research costs can be amortized and the price reduced. In addition, the larger the potential market, the more likely it becomes that a drug company will be willing to do the research and development needed to bring it to market.

Expensive drugs result from small markets or large research outlays. Neither of these conditions is likely to be the case with telomere therapy. The potential market for a telomerase inhibitor to treat cancer is approximately 2 million patients per year in the United States alone.[18] The potential market for a telomerase inducer to treat aging and age-related diseases is more than 100 million people in the United States.[19] Compare this with Pulmozyme, a drug used to treat cystic fibrosis, for which the total market is only 20,000 patients in the United States.[20] Even smaller is the market for Actimmune, a drug used to treat immune deficiencies; the total market in the United States is estimated at only 400 patients.[21] But the market for telomerase drugs will be broad: Neither inhibitors nor inducers will be "orphan drugs." The costs will partly reflect this larger market.

The initial price of telomerase drugs, within the first year or two, will be on the higher end, but will fall subsequently. Price reductions will depend on regulatory and liability costs, but reductions are likely to occur quite quickly as the market widens and as alternative—illegal—sources come on line. Alternative sources are likely to appear in the United States and other developed countries even where patent law is enforced. Just as LSD and many other drugs were produced in college and private laboratories in the 1960s, similar facilities may attempt to produce telomerase agents once the basic process is known. In fact, this is likely to be even more common than it was with the hallucinogenic drugs of the 1960s. The market for such drugs was relatively small; the market for telomere therapy is almost universal. On the other hand, the frequency of use for a telomerase inhibitor or inducer is not as high as it was for hallucinogens. Much more important, however, there was no legal and safe source of LSD and similar drugs in the 1960s. Telomere therapy will have a safe, legal source. There will be little demand for bootleg sources if the drug is cheap and available from a legitimate pharmaceutical source.

Nor could some group suppress the technology or keep it private. Any technically adept laboratory could duplicate the work in a few years. There is little potential for any group or country to hold a monopoly on the techniques.[22]

Research, production, and distribution are not the only costs of marketing a drug. The legal, liability, and regulatory costs have also become major factors in setting the ultimate price to consumers. These last three factors create an additional cost that figures prominently in a few countries such as the United States but almost not at all elsewhere. We charge ourselves this premium in an attempt to guarantee safety and reliability and to permit recovery for damages that would not be considered in many other countries. We don't yet know to what extent these will play a role in telomere therapy.

Telomerase inhibitors, used to treat cancer, will have an advantage over most other drugs and over telomerase inducers in particular. Cancer therapies are held to an appropriately different standard of safety, and even efficacy, by the FDA than are other drugs. They can move more rapidly through the regulatory maze, because of the nature of the disease that they treat. Both patients and the FDA recognize that certain drugs, cancer drugs among them, are special.[23] We tolerate side effects and risks that would be intolerable in, say, an antibiotic. Would you take penicillin if it caused your hair to fall out, weakened your immune system, and made you anemic? Yet, until now, most cancer therapies have had these effects and worse. More often than not, however, they were worth using despite the horrors of therapy, because the ravages of cancer were even more horrendous.

Consequently, the regulatory hurdles are smaller for cancer drugs and the litigation threshold higher. Telomerase inhibitors will have a relatively low non-drug-related cost. They will move quickly into trials and then into clinical use. The liability costs will be relatively small; from almost any vantage point, the price will be reasonable, particularly compared with current costs of treatments that are also less effective.

On the other hand, a telomerase inducer used to prevent or reverse aging—as opposed to a telomerase inhibitor that would treat cancer— will be a therapy in search of a disease. Aging is so universal, so accepted, that it will be hard to gain regulatory approval for its treatment. Yet everyone ages and most will want a drug to prevent and reverse it, so there will be enormous public pressure for approval of such a drug. Still, because aging is not accepted as a disease, the FDA may have trouble approving a drug meant to "cure" it.

As discussed earlier, aging comprises a collection of diseases, any one of which might be considered a legitimate target for FDA-approved therapy. For instance, no one argues that coronary artery disease is not a disease. A drug that purports to treat aging may find the maze impassable, but one that treats heart disease, dementia, or osteoarthritis will have the same chance for approval that other drugs have.

In the case of an eight-year-old progeric, aging is clearly a disease, even in its narrowest definition. A drug that will return health and a stolen childhood to an eight-year-old, who otherwise may die of a heart attack tomorrow or a stroke next month, will clearly be more easily approved. Once that telomerase inducer has been approved to treat an eight-year-old, it can be used for an eighty-year-old.

There are other avenues for regulatory acceptance of a therapy to cure aging itself. For instance, if an inducer could be shown to restore the immunity of an AIDS patient, it would soon become available. If the only accepted use was for treating AIDS, but the technique was effective in treating age-related diseases and even in reversing aging itself, most people would use it, even if it were not FDA-approved.

What about liability costs of a telomerase inducer? How can we tolerate *any* risks in a drug that "cures" something that isn't a disease? Of course, our actions argue that aging is a disease: We will tolerate risks and side effects in such a drug, but to a smaller extent than we might in an official "disease." If telomere therapy reliably reversed aging, but caused universal hair loss, most of us would still use the therapy. If the hair loss occurred in only one person in a thousand, that one person would likely sue and would likely win the case. What if it caused cancer in one in a thousand patients? What if it caused some deaths? We accept these risks routinely in using cancer drugs, but are less likely to tolerate them in reversing aging, a slower, but far more certain route to death than is cancer. Perhaps it is the pace of the disease, perhaps the universal nature of aging that makes us more tolerant of it.

As the risks define themselves, the liability-related costs of the drug will become lower and stabilize, although some liability risks may not become evident for decades, as we will see in the last chapter.

When will telomerase inducers become available to you? Within the next two decades, you will be able to use telomere therapy to extend your life and increase your health. This is a loose prediction, yet remarkably specific considering that in all of human history we have *never* altered the maximum human life span as much as a single year. We can make such a specific prediction because now we finally understand what makes us age, now at last we have the tools to change that. And now, as we near the end of our millennium, we have at last discovered the keys that reset the clocks of aging.

We know that telomerase resets our cellular clocks, but it is available in only small amounts and is effective only for small numbers of isolated cells. As discussed earlier, telomere inducers are being actively sought. Each inducer must be screened for its ability to penetrate into cells and to survive long enough to work, and for its risk of side effects. A drug that rejuvenates our cells but injures them in the process will be of no use to us. There must be a "therapeutic margin"—a dose that is large enough to extend the telomeres but that doesn't cause side effects. Whatever the safe dose, it must enable the drug to penetrate sufficiently into all your cells and to do it quickly enough that your body doesn't destroy, or excrete, the drug before it works.

Given what we know about other drugs and other searches, about the strategy and the resources currently at work, the search for a safe and effective telomerase inducer should take only a few years, about the same amount of time that was required to find a telomerase inhibitor. But will it be effective and safe in a collection of human cells? Our search is the first step; next we have to prove it will be effective and safe for you.

Trials on animals should begin before the year 2000; their purpose will be to determine whether we can take old and sick animals and reverse their aging, making them younger and healthier. Who will be the first humans to try telomere therapy soon after? Will we offer it to progeric children as an experimental therapy for treating what is otherwise a fatal disease? There are few children with progeria, and it will be difficult to prove the drug safe and effective by treating only a handful of patients. But if we want to use it in a larger population, what disease should we treat? We will probably not be able to treat aging itself because of the prejudice against its being called a disease.

The first trials on humans will no doubt involve patients suffering from such serious ailments as heart disease. The first trials will be *ex vivo* studies, in which cells from the vessel walls are removed, cultured, altered (their telomeres reset with an inducer), and replaced; or they will be trials in which we administer the telomerase agent locally to a part of the body. For example, as mentioned previously, we might put a catheter into one of the coronary arteries and flush it with the telomerase agent to reverse the local damage and *prevent* a heart attack. Such preliminary trials will soon be followed by giving the inducer to the entire patient. The studies will broaden to dementias, osteoarthritis, and a multitude of other disorders. New approaches will be tried, new successes gained. The pace will quicken.

We will see telomerase inhibitors before we see telomerase inducers. Cancer will be the earliest and easiest target for therapy. Trials of new drugs toward this end should be in place within the next two years.[24] A clinically effective telomerase inhibitor should be available well within ten years and by some optimistic estimates even earlier. Cancer will be cured at the same time that we are just getting used to the new millennium.

During the next few years, excitement will mount over using telomerase inducers to prevent heart disease, strokes, Alzheimer's dementia, and aging itself, but there will be few tangible results at first. Scientific, medical, and public discussions will focus on the therapeutic possibilities and the social effects of this revolution. From time to time, we will hear of breakthroughs: about the first inducer, the first proof of a safe inducer, the first animal trials. By 2005, the first human trials may have begun, showing that we can successfully reset the telomeres in the cells of your body. Shortly thereafter, and before 2015, telomere therapy will be available to all of us. The most remarkable change in all of human history will have begun.

CHAPTER 7

THE REWOUND
CLOCK

NOR ALL YOUR TEARS

The moving finger writes; and, having writ,
Moves on: nor all your piety nor wit
Shall lure it back to cancel half a line,
Nor all your tears wash out a word of it.

—OMAR KHAYYÁM, *THE RUBÁIYÁT*

TO SOME EXTENT, Omar Khayyám will always be correct. Some things cannot be fixed. Telomere therapy will reset our cellular clocks and prevent a number of diseases, but not all of them. We will cancel quite a number of lines and wash out quite a few words with our tears but not all. We can be optimistic, but certain diseases and genes will remain "written," or, having been "washed out," will reexpress themselves as we live longer.

Three variables will affect how well telomere therapy reverses aging and disease: the patient's age at the time of telomere treatment, his or her individual genes, and the interaction between telomere therapy and a disease. Young people will respond more effectively to telomere therapy than will old people. More accurately, people who have experienced little physiological loss from the natural aging process will respond better than those who have already aged. Telomere therapy will enable the cells to divide longer and to replace lost cells in places where there still are reservoirs, such as in blood and skin cells. When reservoirs have been depleted, the clinical outcome will be disappointing; little change will occur in the aged appearance and function. Organs that do not have reservoirs of their most important cells will never regain what was lost. Telomere therapy cannot extend the life span of missing tissues or organs; it cannot bring back tissues that have been irrevocably lost as you aged. This occurs most frequently in tissues whose cells do not divide, such as the neuron cells of the brain and the muscle cells of the heart.[1] For instance, the twenty-year-old, treated to avoid aging, may defer, or altogether avoid, heart disease, but even with telomere therapy, the eighty-year-old who has already suffered two heart attacks and lost three quarters of her cardiac muscle mass will never regain it.

Imagine the skin tissues of two patients given telomere therapy: One was treated at age twenty before significant losses had occurred and the other received treatment at seventy-five, after having already lost some tissue. The patient treated at age twenty will take longer to lose skin elasticity because the cells were reset and are quite capable of replacing their losses. However, the patient treated at seventy-five may never do as well, because some cell types were probably irrevocably lost. To various extents, this holds true for each organ and system. Some cells are lost as we age, some can never be replaced. Patients treated late in life may approach the full, normal function, but perhaps never do as well as they would have had they been treated earlier.

Another variable is that each of us has different genes, and we age in different ways. But even so, there will be very little difference in how each person responds to longevity therapy. The telomere mechanism that directs aging is universal, not only in human beings but throughout vertebrates, and is almost identical in all multicellular life. At the telomere level, we all age in exactly the same way; the primary mechanism for the institution and timing of human aging is universal among our species and allows for no individuality in its initial expression.

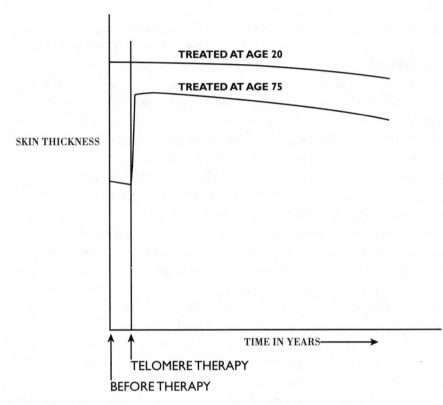

Fig. 7.1

Secondary mechanisms, above the telomere level, are a different matter, however. The telomere may universally control the genes, but the genes themselves differ from person to person. At the clinical level, no two people age in exactly the same way. If longevity therapy can erase and reverse those differences, then it shouldn't make much difference if you age differently from someone else. But if there is anything that telomere therapy doesn't fully reverse, a heart attack, for example, then there will be differences in how individuals respond. If most people fall ill to heart disease only in their sixties, but your genes make you succumb to it in your twenties, then your response to telomere therapy may be disappointing. Even at age thirty, it may be too late for you to have a good result if half of your heart muscle was lost to a heart attack.

Further, although DNA repair is excellent in almost everyone, some individuals show slight differences in speed and accuracy. If an error isn't repaired and remains part of the cell, then neither the error itself nor the damage it causes can be corrected by telomere therapy. Unrepaired DNA damage—accumulated over time—is just one example. The efficiency of our defenses to protect us against entropy varies from person to person. Some of us are better at repairing DNA than others, and some of us trap free radicals better than others. Individual aging is partly luck—the result of how often we encounter random damage—and partly genetic differences in how we repair the damage we encounter.

Although some of us have better defenses than others, no one's defenses are perfect. In sum, no matter how effective are our secondary mechanisms, some damage will accumulate over a long enough time, and we will slowly age regardless of telomere therapy. Individual genetic differences will express themselves in our individual rates of aging even with optimal telomere therapy. You will accumulate damage; entropy will remain a challenge and an enemy.

In spite of this note of realistic pessimism, telomere therapy will have profound and positive effects on your life span and on the diseases that are the expression of your aging. Although some loss cannot be reversed, other facets of aging—metabolic changes and most skin changes, for example—are likely to be quite preventable or reversible. The following sections will explore the medical effects of aging on each body system, progressing from those in which optimism is warranted, through those in which only a cautious optimism is appropriate, to those in which the results are likely to be disappointing.

W H A T   W E   C A N   C U R E

All truth passes through three stages. First, it is ridiculed. Second, it is violently opposed. Third, it is accepted as being self-evident.

—ARTHUR SCHOPENHAUER

We have two sources of information for predicting what telomere therapy will prevent or reverse: our knowledge of the mechanism of disease and our knowledge of premature aging, such as occurs in Hutchinson-Gilford's progeria.

The origins of some diseases are strongly affected by the telomeric clocks in our cells, and will therefore be affected by longevity treatments. Other diseases that are independent of the aging cascade are unlikely to be as affected. For example, the loss of your "permanent" teeth probably results from wear and tear, and is only distantly dependent on the state of your telomeres. This independence holds not only for the cells in your teeth, but those in your gums, salivary glands, and immune system. These cells, and their telomeres, certainly play a role in how strongly built or well protected from decay your teeth are, but for most of us the longevity of our teeth is more a matter of hygiene, diet, and professional care than telomere loss.

Based on what we know about how the body works, we could continue to extrapolate about how various diseases will be affected by longevity therapy, and our conclusions would be reasonably accurate. However, only after we have tried longevity theory will we know for certain what works and what doesn't. Still, most of us would like to acquire some idea of what we might be getting into. Is there any better way of estimating what longevity therapy will be able to do than just extrapolating from our knowledge of aging and disease?

One way of determining which diseases will be affected by lengthening the telomeres is to ask what happens when the opposite occurs, when the telomeres are too short, which is what occurs in progeria. The progeric syndromes, particularly Hutchinson-Gilford, provide a view into what happens when the aging cascade is accelerated and, therefore, what diseases are closely dependent on the telomere. Rapid aging in progeria sheds light on "age-related" diseases by telling us which of those diseases are most likely to be prevented if we lengthen the telomere. If a disease occurs earlier or more frequently when the telomere is too short—as it is in progeria—then we might be able to delay the onset of that disease, or to prevent it altogether, if we can relengthen the telomere.

Though such a conclusion is tempting, we still can't be sure that just because "age-related" diseases—such as heart disease and strokes—occur early and frequently in progeric children, they can be altered or prevented by telomere therapy in those who age normally. Perhaps the fact that, in progeria, aging is occurring in a child—and much faster than normal—alters the course of the "age-related" diseases that they suffer from in unexpected ways. Nevertheless, taking progeria into account probably improves our guesswork.

What will happen to a disease that is accelerated in progeric children after we use telomere therapy? Pessimistically and realistically, the disease might still occur, though more slowly, once we stop or reset the telomeric clock. And even if it is preventable, it still might not be reversible once the person has it. On the other, more optimistic, hand, relengthening the telomeres might prevent the disease from occurring at all. It might also be totally reversible as well as preventable. A number of diseases are probably preventable if we can relengthen our telomeres, and much of the damage that occurs with disease is probably reversible.

What do logic, a knowledge of telomeres and disease, and progeria predict will be changed when we lengthen your telomeres? Children with Hutchinson-Gilford progeria live at most about two and a half decades, but most die before they become teenagers. Some would say that they die of old age or short telomeres, but more simply they die of heart disease and strokes. The typical child with progeria has severe coronary artery disease and vessel disease in general. They are bald and have thin, translucent skin, no significant fat layer, and "age" spots. They sometimes have osteoporosis and arthritis, but they don't have cancer or Alzheimer's dementia.

We don't see more cancer because they don't live long enough to develop significant tumors, and the very nature of their disease prevents most cancers. Before we ever find a tumor—which might take a decade or two to become clinically apparent—the progeric child dies of a heart attack. Even fast-growing tumors may not beat other causes of death. Perhaps even more important, the telomeres are so short in progeric children that only rarely can a precancerous cell survive long enough to become a single cancer cell at all; they die before they ever manage to express telomerase.

The reason that progeric children don't develop dementias is less certain. While cancer and heart disease both tend to manifest in normal aging in the forties, fifties, and sixties, Alzheimer's dementia takes much longer to develop, with symptoms seldom present before the seventies and often still not appearing until we are well into our nineties.[2] This additional three decades or so that it takes for Alzheimer's to develop is probably too long for progeric children. They simply don't live long enough to succumb to Alzheimer's.

There are other diseases—common in progeric children—that will certainly be preventable by telomere therapy. Most prominent is vessel disease, which is caused by cellular aging. Cells that line the vessels lose telomere length; heart attacks, congestive heart failure, strokes, hypertension, aneurysms, varicose veins, and endless sorts of peripheral vascular disease are the result. All are potentially preventable and largely reversible by relengthening the telomeres.

DISEASES OF THE VESSELS

Heart attacks may be prevented if the cells lining the vessels are still capable of dividing normally, as they would be with longer telomeres. Even so, a heart attack could still be caused by an infection of your pacemaker cells, a genetic predilection to form clots that then migrate into one of the smaller arteries of the heart, or trauma to the vessels or the heart itself. Neither infection, deficiency diseases, genetic mistakes, nor trauma will be erased by telomere therapy. And there will probably still be local plaques that can close a coronary artery and cause a heart attack if there is high enough cholesterol or blood pressure, or viral damage to the vessel wall. Telomere therapy removes only one major cause of vessel disease, a cause that plays a role in most of the other causes as well; it does not guarantee healthy vessels, just younger vessels. The chance of a heart attack would fall, but not to zero.

The same will be true of strokes, which should certainly be preventable with telomere therapy. Although young people can have strokes, it usually takes cocaine use, major trauma, or unusual clotting-factor genes. Strokes won't be totally prevented by longer telomeres and "younger" cells, but the chances of them occurring will be less no matter what one's age. However, though we may be able to prevent both heart attacks and strokes, we won't be able to reverse either. Once heart muscle or neurons have died, they are gone forever.

High blood pressure is more complex, and the contributions made by aging cells are subtle. However, it is likely that most of the factors that contribute to the onset of hypertension with aging—such as diminished capillary volume, renal changes in blood flow, elasticity changes in the vessel walls, plaque deposition, and changes in the function of your heart muscle—ultimately result from telomere shortening and will be treatable.

As the capillary bed shrinks, leaving cells with a tenuous supply of oxygen and nutrients, some organs, especially the kidney, compensate by attempting to raise the blood pressure to ensure their own adequate blood flow. The kidney does this both by controlling fluid and salt balance and by sending hormonal messages to the heart and vessels. As the telomeres of endothelial cells shorten, the cells become progressively poorer at recycling the proteins and other molecules that give strength and elasticity to the blood vessel. Plaques are encouraged as the cells lose their ability to cover the innermost layer of the artery. All of these factors play a role in causing hypertension, and each may be prevented if your telomeres are lengthened. Of course, hypertension could still occur; blood pressure is also affected by genetic errors, diet, exercise, injury, infection, diabetes, and other problems, which interact no matter how long your telomeres are.

Aneurysms are a disease afflicting old cells. As we have seen earlier, the weakening of the arterial wall that occurs in aneurysms is found only where cells have almost no telomere left. Most aneurysms can be prevented by permitting the cells to divide and function normally again; longer telomeres will yield younger cells and fewer aneurysms. But aneurysms will still surprise us, striking unexpectedly; they can result from genetically peculiar arteries, excessive stress placed on an otherwise innocent and small aneurysm, or a head-on collision at eighty miles an hour.

As your circulation decreases with age, it affects not only the kidney, and hence blood pressure, but all other organs as well. The endothelial cells that make up your capillaries can no longer replace their daily losses and are unable to maintain the vast infrastructure that supports every cell. The breadth of your capillary bed decreases. Cells that were once positioned near a reliable supply of oxygen and nutrients are now—as capillaries die off and are not replaced—lost in a cellular hinterland, their oxygen marginal, their nutrient supply haphazard and intermittent. As your circulation withdraws, your peripheral cells are increasingly at risk; infections increase, sensation decreases, function is lost, the skin becomes a frail barrier. Telomere therapy can give the capillary cells the ability to divide again, letting them branch out as they had before and resupply distant cells and tissues.

Heart failure, like hypertension, is a disease of many sources and, like heart disease, is a misnomer. Heart failure is only partially a disease of the heart; it is just as much a disease of lost capillary beds and inelastic arteries, whose aging force the heart to do more work for less pay: It has to pump harder while its own blood supply decreases. Once again, the real culprit is the vessels; whether in the arteries of the heart or of the kidneys, there is a growing loss of capillaries and changes in the artery walls. And no matter where these events occur, aging cells are contributing to the heart failure. And once again, using telomere therapy on your aging cells will be likely to prevent and reverse heart failure.

Vascular diseases—heart disease, strokes, high blood pressure, aneurysms, peripheral vascular disease, and heart failure—will be among the first targets of telomere technology. Telomere therapy promises to be most effective in combating aging vessels, and to prevent and to a large extent reverse many of the clinical diseases that result from aging vessels. If telomere therapy offers us only that, it will be sufficient, yet it suggests great potential for success in other areas as well.

ARTHRITIS

Of the two forms of arthritis, rheumatoid arthritis, roughly speaking, is a disease of the immune system, while osteoarthritis—also called degenerative joint disease—is a disease caused by overuse. Rheumatoid arthritis has been blamed on bacteria (including tuberculosislike organisms), viral infections, and autoimmune disease, each of which destroys the joint, causing inflammation and pain. No matter what triggers rheumatoid arthritis, its engine of destruction is the immune system. The cells in the joint are damaged, signaling an immune system overeager to attack. Inflammation ensues as the immune system overreacts and the joint is destroyed. If rheumatoid arthritis responds to telomere therapy, it will not be because of any direct effect on the cells of the joint, but because the immune system becomes more accurate with telomere therapy. This mechanism is more indirect than that which is likely to occur in the case of osteoarthritis (and so will be discussed in the next section).

Osteoarthritis is thought of by many people as a natural consequence of aging; the joint surface, after too many years of being crushed, is finally destroyed. The joint loses its smooth cartilage "bearings" and wears through to coarser bone. No longer able to slide, turn, and rotate, the joint becomes inflamed and its every movement is painful.

Shortening of telomeres most likely is at the root of osteoarthritis. The cells of the joint lose the ability to divide and replace themselves; the more often a joint is stressed, the more the cells are called on to divide and replace lost joint cells. Joints that are used the most degenerate fastest, and ultimately their cells will have the shortest telomeres. Those aging cells become less efficient at replacing the proteins that surround the joint and give it its resiliency and smooth operation. As this aging process continues, the cells still capable of protein replacement increase production, but it's a losing battle, because the rate of degradation increases faster than that of replacement and cartilage is progressively lost. At the same time, the nutrient and oxygen supply to the joint—tenuous and secondhand even in the best of circumstances—decreases with age. Each of these is due to telomere erosion and is therefore amenable to telomere therapy. Joints will still wear out with sufficient cause, but telomere therapy will postpone the onset, perhaps indefinitely.

THE IMMUNE SYSTEM

The immune system certainly ages, but it also becomes more experienced over time. Like the brain, it "memorizes" a vast number of antigens over the decades and is prepared to battle them. By early adulthood, you are immune to most common childhood viral illnesses; in your seventies, you should be immune to a vast number of common cold and influenza viruses (of course, new strains of viruses the body can't have encountered show up every year, even the common cold, which comes in innumerable varieties). As you age, your immune system becomes both sloppy and ineffective. It may accurately recognize the enemy, but the recognition will be slower and less precise, and it cannot muster its troops the way it once did in your youth.

Older lymphocytes don't divide as rapidly or as reliably as younger ones. They secrete less of several proteins that are critical to an effective and orchestrated response. Internally, they have also changed for the worse; many cells are no longer as capable of ingesting and killing invaders as they once were. Some cells work well, but many don't.[3] Like the cells lining blood vessels, some have been stressed and divided a great many times while others have led a quiet life and divided only a few times. Some lymphocytes have had to divide frequently in order to battle enemies; as they divided, their telomeres have run down, leaving many unable to divide any further. And those that still can, do so too slowly to be effective. Their rate of division gets progressively slower, and the probability of surviving even a common infection decreases. Aging lymphocytes become your Achilles' heel.

Not all of your lymphocytes are old; some have been rarely called upon and have divided less often. Those cells sit with their telomeres unspent, capable of responding quickly and efficiently to a challenge that may never come their way. But even these cells lose their support as you age; they may have been held in reserve, but they depend upon other lymphocytes that *have* aged.

In some ways, telomere therapy will make your immune system better than it ever was. The cells will continue to retain their "memory" of their enemies, but they will also now respond as accurately, quickly, and forcefully as those of a young immune system. Lymphocytes will again divide rapidly and again produce the necessary immune factors. The immune system will have the energy of youth and the experience of age.

But what can't telomere therapy do for the immune system? As in any system, it cannot bring back cells that have died. Suppose an entire line of lymphocytes dedicated to a single enemy was wiped out by a combination of previous battles with that enemy and cellular aging. Telomere therapy cannot bring back the line. If you have other cell lines—you usually do—equally capable of dealing with a threat, you will stay healthy even if you encounter the same enemy. If you don't, you will live with a gaping hole in your defenses, one that could be breached with a single sore throat.

THE NERVOUS SYSTEM

The nervous system is often compared with the immune system. It is an apt parallel, especially with respect to aging. Both systems have "memory" that suffers with age; both systems know a lot, though neither can accurately recall what it knows. The nervous system differs mainly in that its neurons don't divide and don't age; to the extent that aging occurs in the nervous system, it is secondary to aging of the glial cells and the vessels that supply them.

There are, however, exceedingly rare cases in which neurons do divide and do age. These are the olfactory neurons—the smell receptors, whose cells divide and replace lost olfactory neurons throughout your life—but as the cells grow older, and have divided too many times, their telomeres shorten and their ability to divide slows. You have fewer olfactory receptors as you age and a dimmer sense of smell, because of the decrease in receptors' cells.

If we reextend their telomeres, the cells of your olfactory receptors can divide again, repopulating your olfactory mucosa and returning your sense of smell. However, each of these neurons is specialized, so if, for example, you have completely lost the cells that can respond to, say, apple blossoms, you will never regain them. Luckily, you don't have single cells, or even lines of cells, that respond only to a single odor. Rather, you have cells that respond strongly to a few odors, less strongly to others, weakly to still others, and not at all to some. Telomere therapy will likely return to you a much improved ability to smell, but with some unpredictable changes in your perceptions and preferences, as those olfactory neurons that remain, divide anew and signal all the more strongly, while those that are irreversibly lost no longer contribute to the olfactory orchestra.

THE SKIN

Your skin is the place where the effects of telomere therapy will be the most obvious. Our judgments about telomere therapy are generally quite simple until we begin to consider its possibilities for skin and hair; then it becomes important to distinguish cosmetic from medical treatment. Telomere therapy offers us both. Though our skins will look younger, that is insufficient reason to either approve of or disapprove of telomere therapy. Although there is a social importance attached to younger-looking skin, the impetus for undergoing and administering telomere therapy should be to make the skin cells *younger* (and *more functional*), not simply younger looking. Your skin is the outermost aspect of your immune system. Older skin is prone to fungal and bacterial infections, doesn't heal quickly, and easily develops pressure ulcers, occasionally with fatal consequences. Lacerations that take a week to heal in a twenty-year-old may require a month for someone older. The skin of an older person may be so paper-thin that it tears with a gentle fall; it may not be suturable, and it may not ever heal properly. But these functions may be brought back to their youthful vigor and efficiency with telomere therapy.

CANCER

All of the diseases discussed so far in this section may be affected by lengthening the telomere. But there are other diseases in which the cure will be achieved by *shortening* telomeres. Both cancer and parasitical disease can be cured by the selective use of telomerase inhibitors. A telomerase inhibitor can be used to prevent cells from dividing endlessly. If these cells are cancer cells or parasites, they will age and die.

In the case of cancer, a telomerase inhibitor tailored to block the action of human telomerase is used. We have already isolated telomerase inhibitors that prevent the lengthening of telomeres in malignant cells. Because these cells are usually already on the brink of losing their telomeres—their clocks continuously reset to the "eleventh hour"—a telomerase inhibitor pushes them onward into rapid senescence and death. Even in cancer cells, which have longer telomeres,[4] an inhibitor prevents further lengthening.

In 1994, the first example of telomerase inhibitors was isolated by researchers at the Geron Corporation in California.[5] The initial results show that "antisense RNA" is effective against ovarian cancer cells in vitro and has no effect on normal fibroblast cells.[6] Further work is already in progress, both on other types of cells in vitro and on animals with cancers.[7]

Other than cancer cells, there are at least two other kinds that express telomerase: germ cells and a few rare white blood cells. Both ova—dividing only before birth—and sperm cells—produced throughout life—have long enough telomeres to survive while we treat cancer cells with telomerase inhibitors.[8] A cancer cell might have a long enough telomere for only ten divisions once we administer a telomerase inhibitor,[9] while a germ cell might have enough telomere for several hundred divisions. The cancer cells may die in days or weeks, while the germ cells will continue to function normally. A telomerase inhibitor could wipe out malignant cells with little effect on germ cells[10] and almost no effect on the rest of your cells.[11]

What about the rare white blood cells that also express telomerase? We know almost nothing about them. First reported in early 1995,[12] they have not yet been identified. If they divide slowly or have long telomeres, relative to cancer cells, then there will be little to worry about when we give a telomerase inhibitor systemically to cure cancer. But what if they have relatively short telomeres and divide often, having just enough telomerase to survive? What would happen to them if we gave a telomerase inhibitor? These questions—the identity of these cells, their division rate, and their telomere length—need answers before we can understand the risks.

Telomerase inhibition will only work on cancers that use telomerase to continually reset their cellular clocks. Which cancers are those? So far, every cancer that has been examined expresses telomerase sooner or later.[13] But do all cancers express it? Probably, although the answer depends on our definition of a cancer cell. In some precancerous cells, some benign tumors, and some neuroblastomas with a favorable prognosis, there is either no demonstrated telomerase activity or very little of it.[14] Cancers that don't express telomerase are less malignant than those that do. They are also more responsive to current therapy—or even benign neglect—and less deadly than their counterparts.

Will inhibition cure cancer fast enough? Could the cancer grow enough to kill you before the telomerase inhibitor stops it? What if either the telomere is relatively long or the location of the cancer is critical? In some cancer cells the telomere is relatively long; how large can the tumor grow before it kills the patient? Are there cancers that have longer telomeres? Certain childhood cancers might begin with their telomeres "fully wound," and form significant malignant tumors before regressing. Those tumors would still respond to telomerase inhibition, but too slowly. They would require additional treatments, such as surgery or chemotherapy. If the tumor is in a critical location, you can't survive even a small tumor. Your heartbeat, blood pressure, and breathing are largely controlled by the medulla at the base of the brain; even a small tumor there would be fatal. The heart's conduction system controls every beat; a small tumor there would also be fatal. We don't yet know how large a tumor can grow without telomerase, but initial calculations suggest that the answer is about four grams—about a teaspoonful of tissue.[15] A mass of that size—on the breast, colon, or ovary—is not life-threatening, but we can't afford even so small a mass in the medulla or heart. Although telomerase therapy will cure cancer, there will be some cases that still require more than just telomerase inhibitors for a cure.

PARASITIC DISEASES

Telomerase inhibitors may play at least one other clinical role. Most parasites, such as the sporozoans that cause malaria, have telomeres, but their telomere bases are slightly different. For instance, while human beings have TTAGGG as their telomere sequence (see Chapter 3), malaria has TTTAGGG.[16] This extra T base may be just enough to allow us to cure the disease. If we could tailor an antibody, or inhibitor, to this specific telomerase, it would induce aging in malarial cells. The same is potentially true of most other parasites; they may be curable by attacking them not with antibiotics, but with anti-telomerase agents. So far, our treatment of malaria has been disappointing. We have found compounds that work for a while until resistance occurs. We have almost eradicated the mosquitoes that carry it, but they have also become resistant and returned. Even the compounds that work don't do so for everyone or on every type of malaria. Soon we might harness aging itself to cure parasitic diseases that until now have yielded only grudgingly, temporarily, and partially. We will use telomerase inhibitors to force parasites to age and die.

Most of us living in developed countries are unaware of the toll of parasitic infection and death. Malaria alone infects 270 million people, about the same number as the population of the United States. Not only do the top six parasitic diseases account for more than a million deaths a year, they cause suffering in hundreds of millions more and they cause economic problems anywhere they occur.[17] Worse yet, the poverty these diseases foster prevents their cure: The budget for parasite research worldwide is far less than the budget for heart disease in the United States. If we can find a cure—through telomere technology or otherwise—the return may be high. Not only would these areas profit financially and in saved lives, but many more would no longer suffer.

Parasitic diseases, such as malaria, sleeping sickness, river blindness, and dozens of others, are potentially curable because they have telomeres that must be relengthened to survive. Although bacteria don't use the same mechanism—and so aren't vulnerable to telomerase inhibitors—funguses have telomeres and should also be appropriate targets for inhibition. We might yet see telomerase inhibitors that—taken by mouth perhaps—would be capable of curing everything from athlete's foot to life-threatening cryptococcal meningitis without dangerous side effects. Fungal infections are fairly common, causing not only skin disorders, but pneumonia, meningitis, esophagitis, and heart disease. Most are trivial, but fatal fungal infections are the daily fare of most large city hospitals, particularly in patients with poor immune function. Perhaps soon, fungal infections will be forced to age themselves to death.

WHAT WE MIGHT CURE

All interest in disease and death is only another expression of interest in life.

—THOMAS MANN, *THE MAGIC MOUNTAIN*

This section discusses diseases of which we have some ignorance, but whose etiology might distantly include aging cells and which therefore might conceivably be cured by telomere alteration. Or they might not; we won't know until we have learned a great deal more about the disease or until we have attempted telomere therapy.

THE DEMENTIAS

The most important of these diseases is Alzheimer's—the most common of a number of dementias that destroy us as we grow older. None of those dementias, least of all Alzheimer's, is inevitable with aging. There is no clear evidence that they result from aging itself, despite the fact that they are seen only among those who have aged. Dementia almost never occurs before age forty-five, and is still rare before age sixty-five. It is found in only about one in ten people over age sixty-five, and in half of those over ninety.

About 15 percent of dementias are due to vessel disease, which will be preventable by telomere therapy. Another 15 percent are the result of Huntington's disease, Parkinson's disease, infections, malnutrition, or metabolic disorders.

About 70 percent of all dementia occurs in the form of Alzheimer's disease. We know a lot about Alzheimer's, but not enough either to prevent it or to determine if telomeres play a role.

If Alzheimer's was found in progerics, we might infer that telomere therapy would prevent it, but progerics don't acquire Alzheimer's dementia. The reason may be either that dementia progresses too slowly to reveal itself before these children die, or that Alzheimer's dementia is unrelated to telomeres. Alzheimer's might also be a pure neuron disease—it is usually regarded as one when it's discussed—unrelated to anything but the slow machinations of some insidious genetic error that destroys the neuron, its connections, and ultimately the life of the person who has it. If that is true, then—since neurons don't divide and their telomeres don't shorten—telomere therapy will offer little to those who develop Alzheimer's disease except more years in which to become certain they will get it.

On the other hand, perhaps progeric children are spared because the linkage is slower for dementia than it is for vessel disease. Certainly that is true of normal aging; dementia comes on much later in life than vessel disease. Perhaps the short telomeres of progeric children accelerate vessel disease more than they accelerate dementia. Perhaps it takes extra decades to go from aging vessels through glial cell damage to Alzheimer's. It is much more likely however, that Alzheimer's dementia simply progresses—even without vessel aging—from aging glial cells to damaged neurons; a progress that also takes decades to show clinically. Progerics don't live long enough to acquire Alzheimer's.

Work done by Dr. Susan Croll, a senior scientist at Regeneron Pharmaceuticals in Tarrytown, New York, suggests that if we take neurons from Alzheimer's patients and replace necessary trophic factors—and glial cells are normally the source of many trophic factors—the neurons look more normal, regenerate, and survive longer.[18] Can telomere therapy revive the ability of the glial cells to produce appropriate amounts of trophic factors as they did when younger? Would that prevent Alzheimer's disease? People with Down's syndrome, whose immune cells have shorter telomeres than the immune cells of those who don't have that malady, acquire Alzheimer's dementia at an early age.[19] Perhaps the fact that they live longer than progerics allows enough time for aging glial cells to inflict their damage on neurons, resulting in Alzheimer's. If the glial telomeres play an important role in Alzheimer's, it is a role we can reverse.

Of course, we can never reverse the dementia and retrieve the mind that was lost. It is difficult to foresee how we could ever bring back a lost personality. Someday, we might add new neurons, but they would not have the complex connections the original had, and they would not revive the person who was lost. The "soul" cannot be replaced. A personality might blossom again, but it would be a new person.

Prevention is another matter. Assume for a moment that Alzheimer's disease, like vessel disease, has many causes, but that at the root of each lie shortening telomeres. We might envision a large role for genetic factors. Alzheimer's is clearly correlated with certain genes—particularly with an apolipoprotein E4 gene—but it can still occur without the gene and be absent in those with it.[20] Sometimes Alzheimer's runs in families, sometimes it doesn't.[21] Despite the genetic predilection, aging glial cells—paralleling the role of endothelial cells in vessel disease—probably play an important role in triggering and contributing to Alzheimer's dementia. Other genetic factors may not be enough to cause Alzheimer's disease independently, or they might do so, but only many decades or centuries later if we can relengthen the telomeres.

This does not conflict with what we know of Alzheimer's disease. Although it remains only a *possibility*, telomeres might be the trigger and telomere therapy might prevent dementia. It may be that aging vessels and especially aging glial cells cause the damage to the neurons that we witness as Alzheimer's. The glial cells age and stop producing trophic factors, the neurons respond by altering their own production of various proteins,[22] and the neurons finally degenerate and die.

If this is true, then Alzheimer's should yield to telomere therapy. But if it is true, shouldn't Alzheimer's dementia be universal in the elderly? Neither heart disease, vessel disease, osteoporosis, nor immune dysfunction are universal in the elderly. To the contrary, there is a lot of variability in aging systems. One person may have severe heart disease, but may have normal joints; another may have crippling osteoarthritis, yet no heart disease. Aging may be triggered and enforced by the telomere, but its expression is variable and depends on your genes. Or, as the progressive increase in dementia with age suggests, it may be universal in those who live long enough to acquire it. Most elderly die of something else first. We certainly have no reason to think that telomere therapy shouldn't help.

There is reason, however, to be more pessimistic about at least one sort of dementia. Robert Sapolsky, an associate professor at Stanford University, wrote a book called *Stress, the Aging Brain, and Age Mechanisms of Neuron Death* in which he made a convincing case for stress as a cause of dementia. Sapolsky showed that neurons in the hippocampus—an area of your brain crucial for memory—die when you are stressed. Stress causes your adrenal gland to secrete steroids that put these cells at risk. During times of stress, when your stress steroid levels are high, even a small additional stress, such as low blood sugar, low oxygen, etc., can kill these brain cells. The hippocampal cells are, in turn, part of the circuit that turns off your adrenal gland's stress response, so the more stress you experience over your lifetime, the less quickly you can turn off your response to it, and the more damage is caused. A vicious, albeit slow, cycle ensues. Over time, you lose neurons and over time your risk of dementia increases, all because of stress.

Nothing about this stress mechanism, if Sapolsky is correct, will likely be changed by telomere therapy, unless the surrounding glial and vessel cell aging contribute to the process. There may be neuron death due to stress alone, independent of cellular aging, and if so telomere therapy is irrelevant. On the other hand, although there is neuron death due to stress, your telomeres—in glial and vessel cells—may contribute to the problem, accelerating the process as you age. If that is so, then telomere therapy would prevent or at least delay the problem. Currently, there is no way to tell which is more likely.

The bottom line for dementia—and especially Alzheimer's dementia—is that there is room to be optimistic, but the question is still open and our ignorance great. The odds are perhaps fifty-fifty in some opinions that we can prevent Alzheimer's, somewhat higher in my own.

OTHER CONDITIONS

There are other conditions whose response to telomere alteration is also still uncertain. For instance, rheumatoid arthritis—as opposed to osteoarthritis—will respond to telomere therapy only to the extent that improving the accuracy of the immune system decreases inappropriate inflammation. As the immune system improves with telomere therapy, becoming more selective in its damage, as it was when it was younger, rheumatoid arthritis might resolve.

Menopause is probably not related to the aging of cells and will remain unaffected by telomere therapy, but we don't actually know. Most of the gynecologic literature favors the idea that there exists an independent clock that counts ovulation and total estrogen[23] exposure over your lifetime—not cell divisions and telomere length—but our knowledge of telomeres is new and not reflected in the previous literature. Menopause is probably timed in the hypothalamus, a thin ribbon of tissue in the center of the bottom of the brain, just behind and above the throat, neurons there calculating the body's estrogen exposure over decades of ovulation. Each woman has a lifetime limit, the product of how much estrogen she produces each month multiplied by the number of menstrual periods she has had. In addition, the ovaries—which begin life with far more eggs than will ever be needed—use up eggs at an increasingly furious pace each month until none remain at menopause. We aren't certain how these two clocks interact; however, although they are possibly tied in some way to the telomeric clock, the odds are against their interacting with the telomere at all. But the rate at which ova are depleted may be determined by the age of the cells that surround and support them—similar to the effect glial aging may have on the health of your neurons. If that is true, then telomere therapy might slow the rate at which ova are used up and thereby delay menopause.

Osteoporosis is closely linked to menopause. With perhaps a decade's delay,[24] it correlates so well with estrogen levels—and to a lesser extent exercise, calcium intake, etc.—that estrogen replacement[25] is probably more effective than telomere elongation would be. Therefore, based on what we now know, the answer to osteoporosis is still hormonal therapy, diet, and exercise rather than some kind of telomere therapy. However, if we do find that osteoporosis is partially due to aging in your bone-forming cells, the osteoblasts, telomere therapy might alleviate the problems it causes. We see this as a possibility because in adult onset progeria, Werner's syndrome, not only does aging begin decades earlier than normal, but so does osteoporosis. That may be because the telomere abnormalities in Werner's patients bring on menopause earlier and menopause brings on osteoporosis, but it may also be a direct effect of telomere shortening on osteoblasts.

Adult onset diabetes, in which the patient usually does not require insulin injections, is also found in Werner's syndrome. If this diabetes occurs because cells become less responsive to the insulin produced by your body as they age, then telomere therapy could cure the problem.[26] And if most of the problem lies with cells that age secondarily—such as muscle[27]—then once again, telomere therapy could cure the diabetes as it reextends the telomeres of the primary aging cells—such as those in the vessels supplying the muscles. Much of adult onset diabetes has even been blamed on the lack of exercise in the elderly. A general increase in health and well-being with telomere therapy might lead people to exercise more, which in turn might cure the diabetes. On the other hand, if adult onset diabetes is due to the irrevocable cell loss—of the cells that produce insulin, for example—telomere therapy will not be effective.

Other possibilities for telomere therapy include preventing macular degeneration (a form of blindness due to retinal disease in the elderly), hearing loss, and other forms of vision loss. Cataracts are probably unrelated to cell aging, but we aren't sure.[28] Changes in focal length—visual acuity—may partially result from cell aging and would therefore be amenable to telomere therapy. For the many diseases of aging, there is much to wonder about and very little to indicate whether or not they will respond to telomere therapy. We don't know which of dozens of diseases are partly the result of aging cells—with their shortening telomeres—and which are due simply to cell loss and cell damage from prolonged use.

Telomere therapy has three further possible applications, though they are not clearly related to normal aging. The first, the treatment of AIDS, has been referred to in previous chapters. If the data continue to support the possibility, then telomere therapy might be used to reconstitute the CD4 lymphocyte pool in AIDS patients. Although that would not cure the infection, it could put it into remission. Telomere therapy might do little for HIV infections in other types of cells, such as neurons, but it could save the AIDS patient from infection and early death.

Second, we might be able to grow cells and tissues to order. Using cultures treated with telomerase, we could grow endless cells for clinical replacement. One of the major barriers to culturing cells is that they age as they multiply in culture. To harvest enough cells to be useful, they have to multiply many times, and after enough generations their clocks run down and they stop dividing. However, if we can find a way past this barrier, we could culture yards of skin to graft onto burns, regrow the cells that produce insulin and cure your diabetes, and even have organs that are made of cells from the patient's body, without the problems of tissue matching and rejection.

The third possibility is that telomerase may allow us to regenerate tissue. Unpublished work suggests that many animals that are capable of regeneration may also express telomerase in their normal tissues or in tissues that are regenerating.[29] If that is true, then perhaps we will be able to regenerate lost limbs and repair spinal cord damage that currently lies beyond our abilities.

WHAT WE CAN'T CURE

All the king's horses and all the king's men
Couldn't put Humpty Dumpty together again.

—MOTHER GOOSE

The list of what telomere therapy cannot do is even longer than the remarkably long list of what it can do. That is not surprising because most of our health problems are not the result of aging. Aging is not responsible for malnutrition, infections, trauma, genetic diseases, psychiatric illness, or any of a thousand other individual diseases. Some of these ailments are caused by an irretrievable loss of cells, not a loss of youth. Sometimes an immune system is unable to meet the challenge of a particularly nasty bacteria or virus; sometimes the problem is a lack of food, or severe trauma, or a dangerous gene. Longer telomeres can never make up for missing cells, poor food, neglected inoculations, unharnessed safety belts, or an ineffective genome.

Of the long list of diseases that telomere therapy can't help, most are due to cell loss (the "Humpty-Dumpty effect") or to faulty genes (not short telomeres). Humpty-Dumpty effects—from diseases that involve loss of irreplaceable cells—are fairly common. After a heart attack, for example, a certain amount of your heart muscle—worse yet, of your conducting system—is lost. These cells don't divide and don't replace themselves, so altering the telomere will not make up for their loss. Once your vessels block off and you have a heart attack, you will never get back what you have lost. However, telomere therapy will give you better function out of what you have left, which would certainly lower your risk of having a second attack. On the other hand, you might end up with a body that—although otherwise fit and in excellent health—will always have shortness of breath and chest pain.

The damaged liver of an alcoholic can repair itself, to a degree, but after a point, the liver may no longer be able to replace lost cells and regain lost function even if you do stop drinking. Telomere therapy will probably extend this limit somewhat, but not infinitely.

The same is true of emphysema. The cells of the lungs are capable of some degree of division, but they are not able to replace the *structure* of the lung once it is gone. It is as though your lungs were a huge, complex building that tobacco gradually dismantles. If all you have lost is paint and furnishings, then telomere therapy will probably restore most of the function. But once you have taken down the walls and girders, the remaining cells—even if they have long telomeres—will never re-create anything that resembles a functioning structure.

This also holds for damage and trauma, which includes everything from losing your leg, to the loss of your "permanent" teeth, to changes in the lenses of your eyes resulting from ultraviolet exposure. If the framework is gone or an organ is missing, and there are no cells to replace the loss, telomere therapy won't help.

Telomere therapy's ineffectiveness against the Humpty-Dumpty effect is only a small part of what it can't do. Telomeres don't make up for bad genes. "Bad genes" is a curiously naive misnomer but a useful category; no gene is bad except in the context of your other genes, and also of your entire environment. Some genes are dangerous when left to themselves, but useful if there's another gene they can work with in tandem. Some genes are dangerous in one environment, but may save your life in another. Genes don't act individually; they act in the total context of the organism—all the cells, all the other genes, all of the environment. A more apt concept than "bad genes" might be a "bad gene mix" or even a "gene/environment mismatch."

Whatever the label, certain diseases are plainly due to genetic inadequacies in the context of your environment. Whether these are complex genetic interactions or simply the result of a single disastrous gene, the blame for many diseases does not lie with the telomere, but with what is between your telomeres: millions of genes, most of them useful, but some fairly nasty and dangerous. Those genes cause or contribute to diseases that will never be cured—or in some cases even altered—by telomere therapy.

These diseases include not only the ones we commonly recognize as genetic afflictions, but bacterial and viral infections, immune and autoimmune disorders, and most common psychiatric illnesses. Although, as we have already discussed, telomere therapy can improve your immune function, we need to be clear in this section about what it cannot do. It cannot make your immune system do what it wasn't designed genetically to do. If your immune system is prone to allergies, it will continue to be. If you are prone to autoimmune disease, for example, multiple sclerosis, you will continue to be. If the immune disorder is independent of the aging of your immune cells, it will not be altered by telomere therapy. None of the problems that result from "bad genes" and consequent inadequate or inappropriate immune function, such as psoriasis, irritable bowel disorders, bacterial infections, viral infections, and a hundred other conditions, will be improved by telomere therapy. Telomere therapy cannot cure most infectious diseases or most autoimmune diseases. In some particular disorders, for example trisomy 21, the immune system may malfunction solely because of short telomeres and in such cases telomere therapy will be effective.

Our previous discussion suggested that we might use telomere therapy to cure fungal and parasitic infections, but even if that is successful, it provides no leverage toward killing bacteria and viruses that do not have telomeres or telomerase. Thus telomere therapy may help us cure athlete's foot or malaria, but, other than making your immune system younger, it won't help us to cure a strep throat or the common cold. These organisms cannot simply be killed by using telomerase inhibitors as we might in the case of yeast infections and malaria. Even a healthy, youthful, and experienced immune system has weak points.

Almost all genetic diseases, with the exception of progeria,[30] are independent of telomere length, and therefore will be unaffected by telomere therapy. Genes will not be rewritten just because we reset the cellular clocks. Included in this long list of genetic diseases are cleft palates; congenital heart defects; sickle-cell anemia; muscular dystrophy; esoteric metabolic deficiencies, and cystic fibrosis.[31]

Psychiatric illnesses are largely genetic, but the ongoing discussions of nature versus nurture show how complex and ill defined they are. What we do know is that little of the blame for most of those illnesses resides in your telomeres. However, a few psychiatric problems—depending on how loosely we define the term psychiatric—can be attributed to cellular aging, among them a few types of depression. But most cases of depression, psychosis, schizophrenia, and dementia—Parkinson's, for example—are probably completely independent of cell aging.

Dietary deficiencies also cannot he helped by telomere therapy. Whether starvation or simply a mild deficiency of a single vitamin or mineral, none of the diseases caused by the lack of proper nutrition will be improved by lengthening the telomere.

Other things are also likely to be independent of the telomere. For instance, baldness is probably determined by a genetic timer that turns off hair growth when it has seen enough testosterone. Men differ in how their timers are set but, those timers are probably unrelated to cellular aging and telomere lengths.

Telomere therapy offers us a great deal, but it will not provide a cure for all the suffering we endure and it will not make us better, or saner, people than we are now.

■   ■   ■

HITTING BY MISTAKE

"Supposing we hit him by mistake?" said Piglet anxiously.
"Or supposing you missed him by mistake," said Eeyore. "Think
of all the possibilities, Piglet, before you settle down to enjoy
yourselves."

—A. A. MILNE, THE HOUSE AT POOH CORNER

Any drug has multiple effects. For example, penicillin kills certain bacteria—the few that are still susceptible these days—by interfering with a single step in making bacterial cell walls. When the wall fails, the bacteria die. But of course, penicillin does many other things. If a small amount of penicillin is placed on an exposed brain, it will cause a seizure. But penicillin doesn't penetrate into the brain very well, so such a side effect is not a problem. For penicillin, or any other molecule, to have an effect, it need only fit into any one of several million enzymes and change the way that enzyme normally works. It can make the enzyme perform better or stop it from functioning at all. Most drugs probably affect thousands of different enzymes, but although a few of these effects are critical, the vast majority are insignificant. Drugs also affect molecules other than just enzymes, but seldom will the effect be as profound and widespread as when it alters a critical enzyme that you, or the bacteria that invade you, depend on.

All drugs have intended effects, all have side effects, and all have to be screened to ensure that the side effects are harmless enough to allow the drug to be used at all. There is almost no way to predict all of the side effects of a drug that lengthens the telomeres, but we can suggest a few and sort them into categories of risks.

The drug would have to affect gene expression—indirectly and perhaps directly as well. If we lengthen the telomere, the pattern of gene expression changes to make the cells act young again. This indirect change in gene expression, however, isn't a side effect; it's the main effect. What if the drug we use to lengthen the telomere does so by directly inducing your own gene for telomerase to express itself? Any drug that does that might certainly affect the expression of other genes in addition to its main target (the gene that holds the blueprint for telomerase). Your genes control everything in cells, so the side effects could be limitless. A telomerase inducer must be exceedingly precise; it must bind so specifically that it induces production of telomerase and yet affects no other genes. If the drug is an analog to telomerase, instead of an inducer, its risk of directly altering gene expression will be smaller, but it must still be specific in lengthening the telomere without causing any side effects.

Beyond this general caveat, however, a few side effects are special to telomerase. Some will be good—bonus effects as it were—and others bad. Let's look specifically at some of these issues by discussing cancer, stem cells, mismatch problems, and reset problems.

WILL LONGER TELOMERES CAUSE CANCER?

Cancer cells already have telomerase, so they won't grow any better with an artificial telomerase, or a telomerase inducer, than they did before treatment. Extending the human life span with telomere therapy won't cause cancer cells to grow any better. Their clocks will be reset, but cancer cells were already resetting their own clocks by expressing their own telomerase before therapy.

Precancerous cells are another matter. Most of us have an unknown number of premalignant cells that have begun dividing and have not yet reached their Hayflick limits. Normally, almost all of these cells would age themselves to death. Rarely, perhaps one in three million cells, does a cell complete the second mutation necessary to become malignant. When this "sociopathic" cell expresses telomerase, it can divide forever, become malignant, and become a cancer.

Telomerase therapy won't turn normal cells into cancer cells and it won't increase the chance of a normal cell becoming a "sociopath." But it will allow precancerous cells to stay alive and divide. Before a cell is damaged, telomerase therapy won't cause any problem; after it has been damaged *and* learned to express its own telomerase and divide indefinitely, telomerase therapy won't cause any additional problem. Only cells that would otherwise destroy themselves will be problems because telomere therapy will rescue them and allow them to survive awhile longer. Only in this single instance could telomere therapy increase the risk of cancer.

Unfortunately, we are not sure how frequently these types of cells occur. Furthermore, even if we do give them a new lease on life, they should continue to age as they divide, and finally age themselves to death. If that is true, then we must reset our cellular clocks carefully, rather than resetting the telomere for so long a time that precancerous cells have a license to divide ad infinitum. We need to bring our normal cells back from the brink of aging without giving abnormal cells too much room to maneuver.

But why should we worry about causing cancer at all, if we are able to cure it with a telomerase inhibitor? Run-of-the-mill cancer cells live a precarious existence, their clocks always teetering at the brink of the Hayflick limit. A telomerase inhibitor should fairly easily stop those cells from dividing. But what if telomere therapy also resets your precancerous cells—which might otherwise die, since they don't express telomerase—back too far from the brink? Those cells can divide a good bit more, causing tumor growth all the while. They may eventually die when their clocks run down, but their telomeres having been reset, telomerase inhibition won't work as well on them. Telomerase inhibition will hurry the death of normal cancer cells already living on the edge, but it won't do anything for cancer cells that have had their clocks reset by telomere therapy until those telomeres shorten again.

The bottom line is that telomerase inhibitors—and, if necessary, other cancer therapy—might need to precede telomere therapy. Telomerase compounds should be used judiciously and we need to watch for a possible increased number of cancer cells after starting telomere therapy. The amount of risk is unknown; the potential exists, and only time will clarify it.

On the other hand, the incidence of cancer may subside substantially. Much of the genetic damage that precedes cancer is caused by aging.[32] For example, as your body grows older, it becomes less capable of combating free radicals that attack your genes, and less able to repair the damage. Older skin is thinner, allowing ultraviolet light to penetrate farther into your body, increasing your risk of cancer. The way you metabolize some carcinogens may change, allowing them to cause more DNA damage than they did when you were younger. Your body becomes more susceptible to damage, which is less likely to be repaired; the genes are more prone to errors, and your cells are more likely to become precancerous.

Aging increases your risk of cancer. Reversing the aging process at a cellular level will reduce the damage that causes cancer. This "side effect" of telomere therapy would certainly be a welcome one. It might be that the best preventative approach to cancer would be to use telomere therapy and the best treatment approach to cancer would be to use telomerase inhibitors. We may be able to prevent most cancers by lengthening the telomere, and to treat most cancers by making sure it shortens.

GERM CELL EFFECTS

How will telomerase inhibitors that are used to treat cancer affect normal cells that express telomerase? Germ cells include ova and sperm. Ova[33] stop dividing before birth and don't depend on telomerase; therefore inhibitors should have no effect on female fertility. However, the situation is radically different for sperm, which form continuously and rely on telomerase to prevent telomere shortening and cell aging. Treating a male with a telomerase inhibitor will cause the sperm cell telomeres to shorten and sperm cell formation to slow down, with sterility potentially occurring. Worse yet, if a sperm with a short telomere fertilizes an egg, the child might have short telomeres in every cell. Males treated with telomerase inhibitors will need to have their children screened carefully for progeria. On the other hand, if only the production rate is affected—rather than the sperm's telomere length—telomerase might even be effective as a birth control measure.

Neither potential side effect—progeric offspring or sterility—is a problem if the male is not trying to become a father. If he abstains from sex, or either partner routinely uses effective measures to prevent pregnancy, then these side effects will go all but unnoticed. Certainly they are not sufficiently dangerous to preclude cancer therapy. Even if telomerase inhibition were to induce permanent changes in the sperm, males still have the option of donating sperm prior to therapy.

SOMATIC CELL EFFECTS

As far as we know, telomerase is almost never expressed in somatic cells, so telomerase inhibition shouldn't affect the functioning of most cells. As for the few exceptional white blood cells (and perhaps others) that do express telomerase,[34] no one is sure yet what the dangers are. Most cancer cells maintain short telomeres and just barely squeak through life. White blood cells that express telomerase probably maintain longer telomeres than cancer cells. If so, they would do well even in the face of telomerase inhibition. On the other hand, if they divide quickly and if their telomeres are shorter than those of cancer cells, there is a significant risk that these cells may "age" rapidly during cancer treatment. We might even lose them, and whatever special immune function they perform. We need to learn a great deal more about these cells before we will know how real the risk is.

The same risk exists for cells that transiently express telomerase. Perhaps certain cells (for example, crypt cells in the G.I. tract) don't normally do so—and so haven't yet been detected—but express telomerase only when they need to divide rapidly. As they divide, the telomeres shorten, and division slows, automatically turning off the supply of cells. If the body needs more of that cell type, it sends a hormonal signal and the cell expresses telomerase momentarily; then telomerase expression shuts down again, but before it does, the telomere lengthens just enough to allow for several more generations of cells. When we administer a telomerase inhibitor to treat cancer, we might kill off this special set of cells. Or when we use a telomerase inducer, we might force the special cells to divide when they shouldn't. We could, potentially, cause a rare, perhaps previously unknown, disease by using either therapy.

MISMATCH EFFECTS

The problem of therapeutic mismatch occurs any time we rapidly alter the body's function, for example by using telomere therapy. In essence, the problem occurs if one part of the body is still too old for another part. Therapeutic mismatch can even occur during normal aging; if a person's cardiac arteries are old and their muscles still young, they may feel energetic enough to jog ten miles, but have a heart attack halfway through. In general, aging debilitates us thoroughly if not evenly. As we age, we no longer have the vessels, lungs, muscles, or inclination to do the things that constantly delight a five-year-old.

When we reverse cellular aging, some cells undo the damage faster than others. Cells that aged secondarily were slower to lose function, and may regain function slowly as well. For example, although the endothelial cells lining the vessels may become young in a matter of hours or days, damage to the rest of the vessel will take months to abate. If the arteries to the heart are improving—though still almost clogged with cholesterol plaques—but the rest of the body was back to normal youthful function, the patient might be tempted to run ten miles—and might not survive it.

Or suppose that muscle mass is regained and activity increases; both of these would place an added load on the kidneys as they filter blood and make urine, substantially raising the risk of kidney failure. If the reflexes that control your blood pressure lag, the risk of stroke and syncope increases. Perhaps appetite increases, but the colon still has diverticular disease. Or the patient might exercise vigorously—with bones that are still osteoporotic. Strokes, heart attacks, renal failure, hormonal imbalances, fractures, and dozens of other problems may occur if the body is not allowed time to coordinate and adjust to the changes.

Any time the increased work of many organs puts a sufficient and unaccustomed burden on a single organ, a therapeutic mismatch will occur. In order to avoid injury, organ failure, or even ironic death in the midst of improving health, we must anticipate the problem and not exceed the capacity of the most delinquent organ.

A more subtle form of mismatch can occur nutritionally. Our nutritional requirements change as we age from twenty to eighty. Telomere therapy will cause the same thing to happen quite rapidly in reverse. Increasing muscle mass will require a higher protein intake; we will also need more minerals (including common electrolytes like sodium and potassium), vitamins, fats, cofactors, and simple calories. The body also has only minimal stores of water-soluble vitamins—thiamine, for instance. A rapid regaining of mass and youthful function may require large amounts of vitamins for new cells and the increasing metabolic demand. If diet is insufficient or the intestines aren't up to absorbing the necessary nutrients, the patient will become deficient. Scurvy, sprue, kwashiorkor, anemia, marasmus, goiter, beriberi, pellagra, and other forms of malnutrition could become the temporary costs of telomere therapy. Diets need to be tailored to the special needs of rejuvenation, much as nutritional requirements are altered during pregnancy, nursing, and childhood.

Mismatch problems will occur more for an aged person given telomere therapy, and less for someone already young and healthy. They should not be a risk at all for patients being treated for cancer with telomerase inhibitors. Overall, mismatch problems are likely to be minor, but need some thought and care. We cannot expect our bodies to tolerate without incident attempts to make them young overnight.

RESET EFFECTS

Do we reset all of our cellular clocks, even the ones we'd rather not reset? The clock for aging is not the same as the clock for early development so there is no chance of it being reset to childhood. These two clocks are not only different, but entirely independent of each other. There is no chance that telomere therapy will reinstate puberty, menarche, early childhood growth spurts, or childhood behavioral patterns.

If the clocks *were* related, it would be important that we reset them only partway. With some difficulty, we could probably reset them at, say, age forty. The difficulty would be to induce your cells to express just enough telomerase—or to supply them with just enough—and no more. Such exact dosing would be a problem, but not an insurmountable one. Potentially, then, you could decide how far to reset yourself. However, most likely resetting your telomeres fully will bring you to a young adult age—twenty, for example—and no younger.

Although this will preclude the problem of being reset to "zero," another possible side effect of resetting the clocks is that it might activate growth in cells whose clocks had stopped. What if a cell is meant to divide rapidly as you grow, and then to stop? Resetting its clock might allow it to divide when it shouldn't. For example, growth of your long bones, such as your leg bones, occurs only at "growth plates." The cells in these areas divide rapidly, but not smoothly or continuously, as you grow, lengthening your bones as they do. One by one—the exact age depends on the individual bone—they stop dividing, ending bone growth. The cells that do the lengthening not only cease functioning, but are eradicated; the growth plate entirely disappears.

There is good reason to suspect that resetting the clock will not reactivate bone growth, because the cells responsible are long gone. Even supposing that bone cells use the telomere to tell them when to disappear in the first place, they are gone by the time you reach full adulthood.[35]

Another example might be the cells of the breasts; specifically, the fat cells, which make up most of the volume of the breast, divide rapidly in the teenager and then stop. But at all ages, the breast continues to respond to estrogen levels. The lack of continued growth is not due to the cells dying off, but to the fact that estrogen, and other hormones, don't keep increasing throughout adulthood. Breasts are likely to be affected to the same extent by telomere therapy that any other tissue is. They may develop a better blood supply and better cellular support from their fibroblasts as therapy resets their cells, but there is no reason to think they will be any larger than they were during early adult life.

Stem cells might use the length of their telomeres to decide when to differentiate into various cell types. Let's assume that when the telomere gets down to a certain length, the stem cells differentiate into either white or red blood cells. As the telomere shortens yet farther, the white cell differentiates into a specific type of white cell. If we reset the telomere completely, we could run out of normal blood cells because all the stem cells were now "back in the nursery," incapable of making normal blood cells. We would be young, but anemic and without cellular immune defenses.

But the timing of blood cell development has no apparent relationship to the telomere. The telomere is quite long in the newborn baby and almost worn away in the old person, yet both make blood cells adequately. In fact, resetting the telomere will probably prevent problems in the stem cell populations where the telomere has already grown too short (as in older people). Telomere therapy might cause reset effects, but, at least in the stem cells that supply our blood, they will be good ones.

In the long run, side effects of telomere therapy will be few. Most of them are more a question of degree than occurrence. Even those that appear most frightful—especially cancer—will be limited and treatable.

FINAL AGING

The immortal gods alone have neither age nor death!
All other things almighty Time disquiets.

—SOPHOCLES, *OEDIPUS AT COLONUS*

Sixty-five million years ago, in the early morning hours on what is now the Yucatan Peninsula, the world almost ended. An asteroid—a small one as asteroids go, but large for anything it landed on—skipped into our orbit and slammed into our planet. Probably, like most meteors, it smashed into the side of the earth on which the sun was rising, on which dawn was still a few hours away, a dawn that never came. It scarcely mattered to the dinosaurs—or anything else alive that morning—how aging occurred—or whether it did at all. Though life didn't disappear entirely from the earth, a large portion of it did, regardless of the state of their telomeres.

The same priority is true of less momentous accidents. If your car is going ninety miles an hour and you hit a concrete embankment, the state of your telomeres is the least important feature in predicting your life span.

We will be able to change most of the things we call aging. We will reverse or prevent some things and cure others. Some things won't be changed with telomere therapy, though in the future they may be accomplished using some other type of therapy. Still, some things, such as death, will never change.

Life is a series of struggles: building your body in the womb, surviving birth, growing to adulthood. At each stage, you have to go over potentially fatal hurdles. You survive croup, but succumb to the measles; survive the fall from the tree, but not leukemia. You make it through one narrow escape after another or you don't survive at all. You succumb to your weakest link, no matter how effective you were at getting over all the other hurdles. Every test is fatal if you fail it.

Historically, our weakest links have usually been infections. Minor wounds carried tetanus, water carried dysentery; things we ignore today killed our ancestors by the millions. Cholera, malaria, and viral illnesses by the hundreds still kill the poor among us, although those diseases in rich countries are no longer the weak links. Instead, we die of vessel diseases, such as those resulting in heart attacks and strokes, and of cancer. We learn to control, treat, and prevent many diseases, but we never get the upper hand completely.

Final aging is a simple concept that is fraught with unpredictability. If we conquer aging as we know it today, we will still age in some new, less familiar way. If we extend our telomeres indefinitely, we may not acquire the diseases we now associate with old age, but we will still eventually wear out and die.

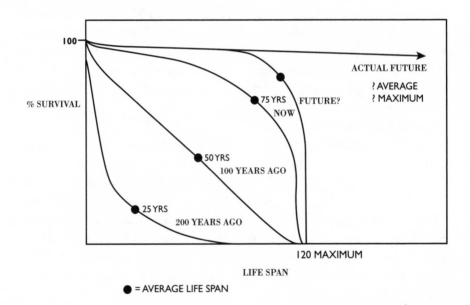

Telomerase therapy alters the maximum life span

Fig. 7.2

The life span curves in Figure 7.2 show that early in human history, most people died young; few made it to middle age, and the average age at death was low. Currently we have flattened the top of the curve; few die young, many survive to middle age, but the curve then drops as it approaches the maximum human life span. Without changing the basic process of aging, the best we can do is to make the curve flatter at the beginning, the angle sharper in old age, and the fall straighter.

If we reverse aging, the curve will not become horizontal. None of us will live forever; the curve will fall, perhaps slowly, slanting downward toward some new "maximum age." What will that maximum age be and what will determine it? What will make the curve slant downward? A number of different processes will cause the curve to slope downward.

Consider accidental death, which is not aging, but certainly causes the curve to slope downward and can be considered one of many "final aging" processes. Accidental death occurs randomly, striking down almost anyone, although it has a predilection for the bold, clumsy, or weak. What would happen to the average human life span if trauma were the only cause of death, if the only things that could kill you were falls, accidents, assaults, and so forth?

Before answering this, three things we must understand about our average life span are its cultural limitations, the age-specific accident rate, and how the question was phrased. The cultural limitations are specific to the year the data was gathered and to the United States: The actuarial data are based on customs and behaviors in the United States at a particular time. A certain percentage of us drove cars or wore seat belts or had bathtubs to fall in; a percentage used guns or ran across the street without looking. All of these figures are accurate for the United States in the mid to late twentieth century, but would be inaccurate decades earlier or later or in other countries.

The "age-specific" accident rate refers to the fact that different ages have different risks. Not many sixty-nine-year-olds drive fast, but they do have slower reaction times, and are less likely to survive an accident than a thirty-nine-year-old. So if we were to ask how long it might take before you had a fatal accident, we would really be asking how long it would take if you forever had the risk of a thirty-nine-year-old, or of a sixty-nine-year-old.

The third thing we must understand is the significance of "average human life span" to the question. Put another way, the question is how long would it take for half the people (the average number) to die? If we began with a million people, how long would it take for five hundred thousand of them to die of trauma? (Technically the last one of those five hundred thousand people to die would represent the median, or average.)

The answer is that if you never aged, but had the body and habits of a sixty-nine-year-old, your average life span would be 693 years. If we are even more optimistic about what telomere therapy can do, and bring your trauma risk back to that of a thirty-nine-year-old, your average life span would be 1,777 years.[36] The point of these impressive numbers is that no matter how high they are, your life span still has limits.

It is, of course, extremely unlikely that we will conquer all disease and be left with nothing but accidents. Once we conquer aging, at least as it is enforced by the telomere, there will still be dozens of other candidates waiting in line to be the next weakest link, from lipofuscin accumulation to mitochondrial damage, cumulative DNA damage, viral alteration of DNA, toxin accumulation, and many more. As we conquer each one, another awaits.

Lipofuscin accumulation is a typical process that may limit our life spans and that may be independent of the telomere.[37] As we age, our heart muscle accumulates lipofuscin to such a degree that it may constitute more than 10 percent of the heart's weight in old age. Although it has not yet been shown to interfere with the functioning of the heart, how far can we push this accumulation before there is nothing left but lipofuscin?

Imagine that you live in a country house that is due to be razed next year to make way for a shopping center. Beside the house is a pit that can hold two years' worth of garbage. By the time it's full, the house will be gone and so will you. Why put time and money into hauling it away when the house and land will be bulldozed in a few months? This shortsighted planning may be exactly why lipofuscin accumulation or any other "weak links" occur as we age. It may not make any sense to our bodies to "haul out the garbage," if the body won't survive long enough for it to make any difference. But will we accumulate too much garbage if we keep the house and live in it for another ten years? All we know is that the efficiency of our defenses against free radicals partly determines how much lipofuscin we accumulate, and that the effectiveness of those defenses is determined by telomere length. So it is possible that extending the telomere will allow us to deal with free radicals as effectively as we did when we were young. And we will avoid lipofuscin accumulation indefinitely. It is also possible that accumulations of other metabolic wastes and toxins will respond to telomere therapy, but there is no way of knowing this until we try it and see.

Mitochondria are the power plants in each of our cells. Without them, we would die immediately. If we lose them over time, they would be another example of final aging. How long can they last? We can estimate the damage rate to mitochondria as perhaps 0.1 percent over your first 100 years, and we can estimate the percentage of damage fatal to a cell as perhaps 70 percent.[38] If these estimates are accurate and if the damage is independent of the telomere, then we could expect to die of mitochondrial loss in about 7,000 years. While that is not a terribly limiting figure, it is not apt to be terribly accurate, either. Cells differ; some have many mitochondria, others few. Some cells have a large margin for error, others a narrow margin. The damage rate is great in some cells, less in others. Mitochondria may divide, but what does that do to their accumulated damage and to their damage rates? Finally, although mitochondria have their own chromosomes (ring chromosomes, without telomeres), they are still dependent upon the rest of the cell, and its chromosomes, for their survival. Perhaps the damage that accrues depends upon changes in gene expression in the cell's nucleus and hence upon telomeres that alter that gene expression in aging. In short, lengthening the telomere might prevent mitochondrial damage.

Tracing the mitochondria backward to conception, we see that they were inherited from the mother. The father's sperm came without mitochondria. Despite free radicals, despite all the possible damage over more than a billion years,[39] the mitochondria you inherit are still working, without any sign of aging—at least not until they become part of somatic cells. Perhaps the "aging" that occurs in the mitochondria in the body is only because the cells around them age. If we reextend the telomeres, mitochondria may not be a limit to either our health or our life span.

Another thing we can't expect is the total repair of all of our DNA, every isomer, and every other error that occurs. Our repairs are efficient and nearly perfect, but only nearly. We will gradually lose irreplaceable molecules to damage and change, no matter what we do to our telomeres. The observation that our germ cell line has managed to survive—despite accumulating molecular damage—for several billion years is irrelevant. Most of these "immortal" germ cells died. It is as though a million people had walked through a mine field blindfolded. The fact that we are the one person that made it safely out the other side doesn't mean the mine field isn't dangerous; it means that we were the only lucky one in a million. DNA damage—mutations—are the mine field and are responsible for evolution. But most mutations are detrimental, even fatal. There has been a savage weeding out process. From each parent we have inherited a germ cell where the DNA damage—the extensive mutation—wasn't quite enough to actually kill it. But if we live long enough, sufficient damage will accumulate to weed out any one of our somatic cells. And if we live long enough, we will accumulate enough molecular damage and loss of irreplaceable cells, neurons for example, to weed us out as well.

Final aging will also occur at higher levels with damage not only to molecules, but to organs. For example, viruses can damage our hearts, retinas, kidneys, brains, and a host of other organs. Their loss will be unaffected by telomere therapy except as it makes our immune system more efficient. Heart muscle may be damaged slowly—but cumulatively—from toxins in cooked meats and kidneys may be damaged by common pain relievers. A thousand substances that we eat daily may be innocuous until we live long enough to discover their long-term danger. We will lose fingers to punch presses, hands to snow blowers, arms to the lumberman's green chains. All of these losses—viral, toxic, or traumatic—are largely independent of the length of your telomeres. Their risks accumulate with years.

Even more difficult to replace, but still potentially replaceable, is genetic and structural information. Not only are our genes present in multiple copies, but much of the genetic information is duplicated in the genes of those around us—relatives, for example. Theoretically, we might be able to replace almost any genetic information that is lost. Structural information, such as data referring to the structure of our lungs or how the nerves connect to our muscles, is also, very theoretically, replaceable. Someday, we could learn to grow a new lung or a spinal cord from scratch. Unfortunately, the information stored in our brains isn't even theoretically replaceable. Once lost, our personalities—what we have learned and experienced, the core of who we are—can never be recovered.[40]

Our boundaries must never detract from what we can achieve within them. We will prevent many of the most serious diseases that afflict us. Many who suffer now, never will again. Cancer will not frighten the generations to come. We can make our lives stronger, healthier, and longer.

CHAPTER 8

TELLING TIMES

INTERESTING TIMES

May you live in interesting times.

—TRADITIONAL CHINESE PROVERB

DURING THE NEXT two decades, we will be able to prevent many of the diseases that undermine our bodies, lives, and minds. We will be healthier and will live longer. We will have the chance to be vigorous and independent. Each of us wants to be healthy, free from disease and pain. This is the promise of the next few decades, a promise that lies tantalizingly close. What will this mean to us, to our world, and to our culture?

Life itself is not always so dear. While disease makes us appreciate health all the more, it is often the opposite with life itself. Those who are happy with their lives tend to value life; while those living in violence, fear, boredom, and misery tend to value it less.

Those who choose to have telomere therapy are not simply choosing to extend their lives but also to forgo disease. Treating disease, you live longer. Opting for telomere therapy will be a matter of choosing not when you want to die, but what diseases you will allow or avoid. It is a matter of your health span, not your life span.

Extending our health span will bring us both health and the time to live more fully, and it holds no qualifications or drawbacks for the individual. We stand to be liberated from many of the things that make us limited and frightened: cancer, pain, inability, dependence, loss of our minds. We stand to grow as individuals and to gain the energy and leisure to do much that we have lacked time for until now.

Will it be equally good for us as a society and a race? Some things will be good, others will not, yet overall it will be for the good, not only for each of us, but for all of us. There is, of course, no certainty in this—we must wait and see it happen. In the meantime, what can we envision of our future? Although it is difficult to predict, some things appear likely. Population will increase, won't it? Probably. Our systems of Social Security and retirement will change, won't they? Yes, but how? Health care, insurance, employment, and family will be affected, won't they? And will it be for the good? In the long run, it will.

Always in history, as advances are made, there are losses, but the gains are usually greater. Slowly and progressively our lives improve— not in everything, but overall. There has always been poverty; there will continue to be. There has always been disease; there still will be. Yet the world improves and will continue to do so. Now, it is about to improve in ways we have long only dreamed of.

■ ■ ■

P R E D I C T I N G   T H E   F U T U R E

DEWEY WINS

NEWS HEADLINE ON THE DAY THAT HARRY S TRUMAN WAS ELECTED
PRESIDENT OVER THOMAS DEWEY

Predicting the social effects of age reversal is much more difficult than predicting the medical effects. Historically, social predictions have almost always been wrong or, at best, right by sheer chance. The problem is that sociology is descriptive, not predictive: The effects of even small changes may be monumental and unpredictable.

Our best predictions are often merely intuitions, and hard to hem into narrow logic. Still, we assume that we can predict the future, in at least a rough way, based on our knowledge of the past. We do a fair to middling job of it when the predictions are cut-and-dried ones, as in, for example, actuarial tables. Society has always been predicated on a few reliable biological assumptions, for instance, that we will age in a predictable number of years, dying at predictable ages of predictable diseases.

The assumption of aging and its effect on the life span not only has been valid up to now, but has been specific. We have based much of our behavior on that specificity: Not only do we die, but a certain percentage of us will die of heart disease, a certain percentage of cancer, a certain percentage of trauma, and so on. The percentages have varied with time as medical care and social conditions have changed. They have varied with location, as we compared country with country and area with area within a country. They certainly have varied among groups of people, whether defined by cultural, genetic, sexual, or religious differences. On the whole, and for each defined period, location, or group, we have been able to make reliable predictions about death rates and causes of death. Reliable information about the medical history of a group has allowed reliable predictions to be made about the future of the group. Our predictions have been accurate enough to plan retirement benefits, health care requirements, and estate needs long before retirement, sickness, or death actually occurred.

Not that many of us have paid much attention to these predictions. In fact, you might guess that very few of us have cared about or were affected by them. You would be half right: Few of us care, but we are all affected. Often unknowingly, we are affected in day-to-day ways by accurate predictions. Most of us are insulated from and ignorant of the effects that predictive data has on our lives. Yet our health costs, our insurance costs—especially life, health, and disability insurance, but to some extent automobile and home insurance as well—our pensions, our investments, and our taxes all depend upon accurate predictions about illness and death.

Beyond actuarial predictions, we all make predictions about our own life spans and the complications and events we expect to encounter. All of these predictions have been based on the biological assumptions that we will age and die in roughly the same way our ancestors have for generations. But the length of the normal human life span may soon become unpredictable. People will die, but we will be less certain about *when* they will die. People will be afflicted with disease, but we will be uncertain how many will and at what ages, and what the diseases will be.

Barely noticeable at first, the inaccuracy of our actuarial tables will begin to be felt as the first telomere treatments for cancer and other diseases take effect. It will grow as we extend the maximum life span. At first, the tables will need to be corrected every year, and the difficulties of prediction will continue for decades, possibly centuries, until we can gradually reconstruct reliable actuarial tables and establish an understanding of disease under a new set of rules.

This may seem no different from medical advances of the past, but it is. There are at least two major differences: First, most "breakthroughs" in the past added only a few years to the life spans of those treated, rather than decades, or possibly centuries, which will be the case with telomere therapy. Second, most past breakthroughs applied to the very small percentage of the population having a particular disease, rather than everyone, as will be the case with telomere therapy.

Our financial world is very much dependent upon adequate predictions. What will happen to loans, investments, and pension funds when life spans suddenly are extended in a quantum leap? All of these are based on predictions about the future. They assume that the human life span and the diseases that accompany aging will be unchanged or will be altered only in a gradual fashion similar to the way in which these have changed in the past.

Before we endeavor to predict in what, admittedly unpredictable, ways society might be transformed by telomere therapy, let's look at when telomere therapy will be available. Shortly after the year 2000, telomere inhibitors will be available for treating cancer[1] and telomere therapy will be available for extending your life span between 2005 and 2015. Although drugs usually take more than ten years to progress from the lab to the clinic, those that alter the telomere may be cleared more rapidly because of their potential for treating high-priority diseases such as cancer and AIDS. News stories about the potential of telomere therapy to cure cancer have already appeared. As these increase, there will also be more discussion about treating other diseases and extending the life span of those now enjoying good health. Other diseases, such as progeria and heart disease, will become candidates for therapeutic trials of telomerase inducers. Despite concerns, there will be a growing belief that the overall effects on our culture will be positive ones.

Not only will we gain health and longer lives, but we will benefit intangibly. Telomere therapy will return to us the chance to wonder again. Although we won't know how long we might live, when have we ever known? The general expectation at first will be that the healthy youthful life span can be extended to several times its current length.

In the short time that remains before telomere therapy becomes available, we need to prepare for the changes that are almost upon us. Leonard Hayflick—who discovered cellular aging—considered the possibility that we might someday extend the human life span and he understood the necessity to begin discussing the implications.

> It is not yet possible for us to perturb the aging phenomenon in humans or to increase our life span. In my view, those who believe that it is possible or about to happen have an obligation to initiate a public dialogue on the question now. Little has been said about the social, psychological, and economic effects of slowing the aging process or extending our longevity. Less still has been said about its impact on institu-

tions such as social security, life insurance, retirement, and health care.[2]

The remainder of this book is an attempt to initiate such a dialogue—about what will happen not only to the population, but to social institutions and the individual. About what will happen to our families; to marriages, divorces, and our children; to sexual roles; to industry and law; to education; and to medicine. And what will happen to our hopes and our dreams, to our religions, our legends, and our ethics. What will happen is ultimately going to be for the good, but there will be growing pains. We will have to assume new responsibilities and acquire new wisdom to cope with the gift we are given, the gift of life.

THOUGHTS OF MALTHUS

Population, when unchecked, increases in a geometrical ratio. Subsistence increases only in an arithmetical ratio. A slight acquaintance with numbers will show the immensity of the first power in comparison of the second.

—THOMAS MALTHUS, *An Essay on the Principle of Population*

The population of the world is about six billion and is likely to double within the next fifty years.[3] In most population predictions, the curve then flattens out. Population growth has already fallen from a high of 2.0 percent per year in the late 1960s to about 1.6 percent per year and is expected to fall further. When we extend the human life span, these predictions will change, but not as much as you might at first guess.

Over the past five hundred years, population has increased dramatically (see Figure 8.1). Like so many other pools, population is determined by two variables, birth and death rates. What if we delay every death for 100 or 200 years? The population could increase by exactly

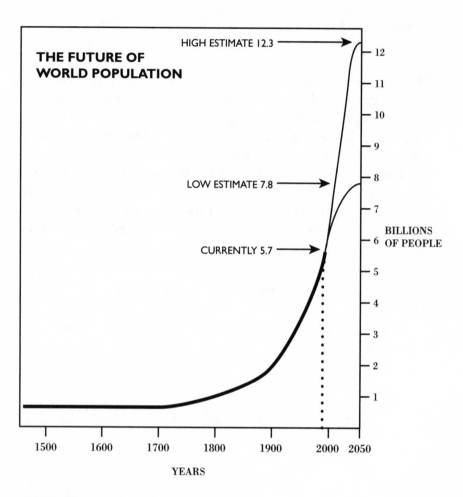

THE FUTURE OF
WORLD POPULATION

HIGH ESTIMATE 12.3

LOW ESTIMATE 7.8

CURRENTLY 5.7

BILLIONS
OF PEOPLE

1500   1600   1700   1800   1900   2000 2050

YEARS

(ADAPTED FROM ROUSH, 1994)

Fig. 8.1

the number of people born during that delay, but that probably isn't what will happen: Many people will still die of diseases unrelated to aging and the birth rate might also change.

Until recently, the concept of a "demographic transition" has been used to explain how population first increased and then leveled off with economic development. As high-fertility, high-mortality nations modernized, death rates fell and birth rates followed with a variable delay that determined population growth.[4] In some countries—France,

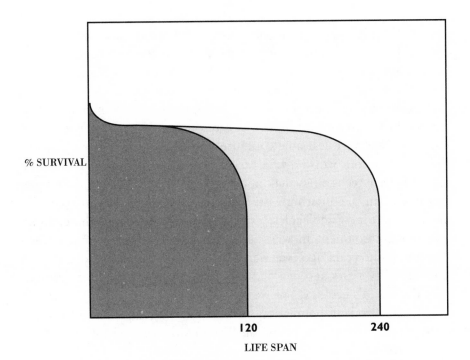

% SURVIVAL

120   240

LIFE SPAN

**If life span doubles, then population (*initially*)
increases almost proportionally.**

Fig. 8.2

for example—the transition took two hundred years, while others—
China for one—required only seventy.[5] Others, like Mexico, are now
in transition. When the birth rate falls to the same low level as the
death rate, the population finally stabilizes—as it has now in most
Western European countries.[6] Telomere therapy will temporarily decrease the death rate, causing a second demographic transition.

The global birth rate will probably be unaffected because telomere
therapy offers little to populations with high birth rates. The highest
birth rates are usually found in Third World countries—for example,
Egypt or Peru—where the most common cause of death is independent
of aging and cannot be cured by telomere therapy. Telomere therapy
promises the greatest increase in health and life span to people in
countries with low birth rates. Sweden, Germany, the Netherlands,
and Italy, for example, have birth rates below replacement—at fewer
than two children per woman, deaths exceed births[7]—and the major

causes of death in these countries are vessel diseases and cancer. Countries with low birth rates will also have the greatest decrease in death rates. Thus telomere therapy will have less effect on population growth than if it increased the life span uniformly everywhere.

Population plays a central role in determining environmental quality, but so does our stewardship of our resources. When the population was small, we were less able to injure our environment, but today our ability to alter our world *compounds* the danger posed by our population size. Modern technology has opened a Pandora's box of techniques that can harm the environment. We now can produce radioactive elements, create new molecules, extract metals, and spread these things into our environment in ways and quantities that we cannot ignore. Five thousand years ago, we were too few and impotent to do much damage. Fifty years ago, we had acquired the power to alter dramatically the world's ecology, but we refused to believe it. Today, however, despite our growing population and our growing capability of causing damage, two factors are acting against this danger: responsibility and perspective.

The environmental movement is only a reflection of something deeper: a growing acceptance of our own responsibility. We are beginning to accept our stewardship of the world, and with it the need to be wise enough and knowledgeable enough to succeed at this task. Environmental laws and publicity are less important than the awareness that we are capable of harming the earth and its inhabitants and responsible for their protection. However, stewardship can only be maintained if the economic ability to do so exists. The poor worry about firewood, the rich about smoke. Developed countries have more pollution than undeveloped ones, but not more pollution per capita. Pollution rates per capita are among the highest in undeveloped countries. Economic development, and the stewardship it engenders, may alleviate the problem.[8] If extending the human life span can improve the economy, it should benefit both the poor and the environment. We may have the economic wherewithal to feed children in Chad and to recycle in China.

Telomere therapy also promises to benefit the environment by giving us perspective. Much of the worst environmental damage occurs slowly over decades and it is difficult to appreciate damage that will occur decades from now. Had you lived two hundred years ago in

North America, you would remember its herds of bison, great flocks of birds, old growth forests, and clean water and air. Knowing that we may live two hundred years should be a new incentive for us to preserve what we still have. If we live long enough, the future will become our home, rather than an ever-expanding landfill. Longer life may enforce what we have only begun.

THE HUMAN OCCUPATION

Can anybody remember when the times were not hard and money not scarce?

—RALPH WALDO EMERSON, "WORKS AND DAYS"

WORKING AND RETIREMENT

We can't work for forty years and retire for two hundred. Someone has to raise food, manufacture computers, and provide the myriad other services we all depend on. We could work and retire as part of a cycle, but we won't be able to retire forever at age sixty-five.

In 1900, the average age at death was fifty, and retirement at sixty-five would have been supportable. In 1935, when Social Security was enacted, the life expectancy was only sixty-one.[9] Now the average age at death is seventy-five; perhaps—with care and forethought—we can still retire at sixty-five. There are still enough of us to support those who have retired. Currently there are about five people working for every one retired;[10] by the year 2030, fewer than three people will be working for each retired person.[11] These figures assume no remarkable change in our life span. What if the average age at death grows to well over one hundred?

Occasionally we think that "the company funded my retirement." The company may have saved it for you, but it was your money. Some retirement plans—for example, the U.S. Social Security system—may even use payroll deductions to pay workers already retired, hoping the plan can stay ahead, like some grandiose Ponzi scheme. The only advantage to the government's retirement program is that it averages out individual differences in life span. Whether you live five more years or fifty, you will still receive a regular—albeit small—check. Many corporations now use "defined contributions" rather than "defined benefits." The company puts money into your pension fund each year; what you receive depends on how much you contributed.[12] Whether you live to sixty-six or ninety-six, you are paid the same benefit. Defined contribution plans make it easy for the company, but chancier for the worker.

Defined benefit plans, on the other hand, are predictable only if the number of workers is large. As long as the average life span is known, then the cost of the benefits is predictable. Unfortunately, even with the relatively minor increases in our life spans of this century, workers have tended to outlive predictions. When we add telomere therapy, no retirement plan can be large enough or far-seeing enough to calculate how much will have to be put aside in a defined benefit plan. A company cannot afford to guess in administering such plans, and if it does, then you can't afford to work for it. Defined contributions will still be viable, but will leave the guesswork to you.

Not knowing how long your life span will be or what diseases will become less common, you will have to take responsibility for your own retirement savings. You might alternate working and "retiring," coming back to a job, or beginning a new one, every few decades. How frugally you live will determine the ratio of work to retirement. I know one man whose ratio now is less than one to ten: He works for one month a year and retires to be a beachcomber for the other eleven. For most of us, however, the ratio is more likely to be four to one or at best two to one: work forty years, retire for ten or twenty.

Historically, retirement—as we think of it today—is a novel concept. The idea that it should begin at age sixty-five was arbitrary— the age has varied between sixty and seventy in various American states and in other countries.[13] Throughout most of human history, people have worked until they were no longer able to. As a child you did what you could, as an adult you had a conventional occupation, until, in sickness or old age, you again—as when you were a child—did what you could and depended on your family to help when you could not. It was one of the major benefits of having a large family and many children.

What are the pressures pushing us to retire or to work longer? Besides our urge to lie back and relax—and our sense of entitlement—there is peer pressure. It has two roots: the urge to advance and the aging of older workers. Each of us wants a chance in the pilot seat, and older workers are not always as productive as younger ones.

In the first case, younger workers want to move up the company ladder and older workers are perceived as being in their way. The older worker has had his or her chance in the position, the younger ones reason, and now the younger worker wants an equal chance. This attitude derives from the myth of the mailroom clerk: "I may be only a mailroom clerk today, but I may be the CEO tomorrow." Although this has happened only in the occasional, improbable case,[14] the dream is crucial and, in a sense, part of our compensation for working. We are paid in prospects as well as in cash. Part of the mailroom clerk's reward is the opportunity to advance. The assistant professor is compensated not only with a salary, but in the currency of future tenure. The new assembly line worker is paid partly in the hopes of becoming a supervisor. We have aspirations, and they are included in what makes a job—indeed, our lives—enjoyable and exciting as opposed to merely tolerable. But what if the CEO stays on for a century, if tenured positions remain filled, and if your supervisor stays almost forever? In an unmeasurable, untaxed, but very real way, your compensation will have been cut. Your chances for advancement will diminish, your job will be less rewarding. On the other hand, if economic growth occurs, there will be more CEOs and more positions to advance into.

The on-the-job pressure for retirement is also rooted in the need to retire older workers as their value declines. Retirement has a value to a business itself and to the economy in general. While some of us become increasingly competent and productive at our jobs, others lose touch with markets, consumers, or technology. And older workers may cost more: They are more prone to sickness and disability; the costs of insuring them reflect these growing health problems. Until now, uniform retirement has provided an easy out when the costs threatened to overrun the benefits.

When we live longer, remaining healthy and avoiding the ravages of age, will we still be useful? Perhaps we will be that much better at the jobs we will have been doing for a century or more. But some of us will grow jaded, or impatient for new challenges and a new career, and others will fall behind and be retired of necessity, no longer able to compete or to produce for the company employing them. If people are forced to retire, it will in most cases be because they have lost their interest, not their health and vigor. On the other hand, many people will grow with their jobs, refining the definition of excellence, becoming career craftsmen who have unmatched decades—perhaps centuries—of experience. We will be old enough to know everything and still remember it.

Many of us change jobs; few of us change careers. But what if you knew you could live another two hundred years? You might become a doctor at age fifty, take ten years to learn to paint, or spend a decade becoming a physicist, a gardener, a machinist, or a cook. Having multiple careers would give us broader backgrounds and perspective, more comprehensive understanding, making us more effective at each career. We could change careers every few decades, using the experience garnered in earlier ones to become that much more adept at those we undertake later. A politician might be that much better for having been a carpenter, a lettuce picker, a teacher, a businessman, an accountant, and a father. A physician might be more understanding and more human for having been a social worker, a policewoman, and an assembly line worker. Currently such career shifts are very difficult to achieve, but they may soon be much easier, or even required. Over the years, many M.B.A. programs have begun to require several years of business experience. Perhaps many training programs in various professions will demand broad, practical backgrounds.

Even if we don't retire, we will continue to save, and we will have more years to let our savings grow. Currently we are afraid that when we retire, our Social Security checks will be too small, our relatives will be overwhelmed, and our health will be too precarious for us to really enjoy ourselves. Even when we live much longer, we will still need to save for rainy days, but perhaps not for the snowy days of old age. We will retire by choice, not because of regulations or physical inability. And prior to retiring, we might take several years of sabbatical for the same simple purpose of enjoying ourselves for which we now take an annual vacation.

ECONOMICS

In the long run, we will all be dead.

—JOHN MAYNARD KEYNES

All of us will die in the long run, but it may be a longer run than any of us planned on. What will happen to our investments, our salaries, our incomes, our taxes, and the cost of living? Will there be an economic bust or an economic boom?

Although the Social Security system begins saving for us as soon as we receive our first paycheck, most of us begin intentionally—and belatedly—saving for retirement only at about age fifty. But if we know we may live a hundred years more, will we still save? Some of us will save if we live longer, most of us still won't. Like the fable of the grasshopper that fiddled all summer, many of us will save only when winter is upon us; those who save will be balanced by those of us who fiddle. Perhaps there will be less investment, in venture capital, business, and research, and more spending; or perhaps there will be more investment.

To the extent that the costs of labor, as opposed to technological innovations, determine the prices of products, we will probably experience an economic boom, because the economy will become more efficient. Labor costs will shrink, and real wages increase. Costs will be reduced for at least two reasons: lower insurance rates and lower training costs. As we lengthen the life span and prevent the diseases of aging, the price of life, disability, and health insurance—particularly in older workers—will fall, as will the cost of Medicare.[15] These decreasing costs will be reflected in a lower cost of labor without any loss to workers themselves.

Training costs will also decrease. It now takes ten or fifteen years to train tool and die workers; and almost two decades for doctors.[16] Extended training periods are common for lawyers, teachers, electricians, plumbers, accountants, nurses, bankers, scientists, and others. It takes years to pay back the money and training hours that have been invested in our lives. Training is a major investment for many companies. Tool and die workers, for instance, may be worth more than the buildings, more than the machines, and more than the customer base.[17]

Labor accounts for two thirds of the cost of production in the United States,[18] and training is a large part of the labor cost. Most workers retire after thirty or forty years; anything that cuts training costs or increases the number of years people can work will reduce overall labor costs. Workers who live—and stay healthy—longer, allow the company to recoup more of their training investment.

Not only will the number of productive years increase relative to training costs, but they will increase compared with other, nonproductive years. The first two decades of life, spent as a child, and the last few decades of life, as an older, retired person, are usually nonproductive, and are paid for by the years we do work. Although the absolute costs remain the same, the relative costs of childhood, training, and retirement decrease in proportion to the number of years we work, causing the cost of labor to decrease. A decrease in the cost of labor lowers the cost of a product, which drives down the cost of living. As labor costs fall, productivity increases, and real wages increase.[19]

This decreased cost is not charged to anyone: It isn't taken from Peter to pay Paul. It derives from having more efficient labor and a healthy work force. And the savings will be returned to everyone's pockets.[20] There will be an unparalleled economic boom for labor and for management, for both white-collar and blue-collar workers[21] that does not guarantee a better life for all, but it is not a threat to income equity, either.[22] At first, some will benefit more than others, and over the next century or so, wealth may begin to accrue to the longer-lived. Twenty-year-olds won't be able to afford a house; sixty-year-olds may have a house and a condominium. The longer you live, the more you can save and the more you will be capable of purchasing.

The effects of population growth on unemployment are unpredictable. The economy and the job market will grow, but so will the number of people seeking jobs; the unemployment rate may decrease as the economy booms or increase as the population does. On the other hand, population increase represents a market increase, and as the market expands, so will the economy.

Even though there are finite amounts of many resources—for instance, real estate,[23] minerals, and timber—and the demand for them will rise, it is difficult to predict what will happen to prices. The real-dollar price of most minerals, for example, has declined or held steady in this century, despite increased demand. The same has been true of food prices, despite an increasing population.

Manufacturing will become more profitable as labor costs go down. The automobile and electronics industries will do better than they would have without telomere therapy as peak earning years lengthen and there are more purchases, per lifetime, of expensive goods. The same increased sales can be expected in the markets for boats, recreational vehicles, and sporting equipment, as well as for golf courses, tennis courts, ski mountains, and the like.

Service industries will increase as demand does. Not only will each of us have more money to pay for services, but the relative costs of those services will fall as training, insurance, and health costs decline for these workers.

Agricultural land will cost more, but balanced against this will be lower costs for labor and technical innovations—genetic alterations of crops, for example. In the food industry, the cost difference between raw and prepared foods—for example, between cocoa and chocolate bars—may shrink as the labor costs become smaller.

Will our longer life spans have the same effect of offsetting the natural rise in the costs of construction and real estate with decreased labor costs? Real estate costs will rise both with population growth and with the *perception* that the population will continue to grow; the expectation of increased demand will drive up prices. Despite the rise in cost, new housing starts will accelerate because mortgage rates will be low, as available capital increases, and because people will have more real income as they save longer and wages rise. The percentage of renters will fall as the percentage of young people in the population falls. Turnover may decrease as people keep their homes decades longer than the current norm; we are likely to see extended occupancy and less employment in this segment of the real estate market.

Shipping, travel, banking, commercial sales, and many other sectors of the economy will burgeon, fueled by lower labor costs and general economic growth. Some of these—leisure travel, for example—will do especially well as disposable income and average age climb. However, banking will see savings shift away from certificates of deposit and other low-risk and low-return investments, into stocks and bonds. The higher long-term return of equities will fit better in our longer investment perspective. If we plan to retire next year, we would be foolish to put all our savings in stocks, but if we don't intend to retire for fifty years, they are a much better investment.

Insurance firms will separate themselves into the quick and the dead. There will always be insurance companies, but the major question will be what to charge. Insurance companies operate by balancing their premiums (the only thing they can control) and their investment return (off your money), against their claims (what they pay when you get sick or die). The change in the actuarial tables will have actuarial departments staying up late with their computers, trying to recalculate the incalculable: How long will you live, how often will you become ill, and with what disease? The good news—for the insurance company, not for you—is that the initial effect will be a fall in the number and cost of claims; the bad news is that we will demand a reduction in premiums, and the companies won't know how to match the two. A side effect of the insurance problem is that those who have invested in annuities and those dependent on insurance payments—for example, the disabled—may be at risk.

Science, education, the arts, and medicine will benefit because the major asset of professionals in each of these fields is their extended, and expensive, training. Science, for example, will benefit from longer retention of teachers and researchers; the downside could be that many young scientists, with fresh perspectives, may find their paths blocked unless an expanding economy creates enough new positions to make up the retention of professionals who would have died off. William Osler—one of the greatest physicians of the nineteenth century—put the issue strongly.

> Take the sum of human achievement in action, in science, in art, in literature—subtract the work of the men above forty, and while we should miss great treasures, even priceless treasures, we would practically be where we are today. . . . The effective, moving, vitalizing work of the world is done between the ages of twenty-five and forty.[24]

But education has always been a squandered asset. Institutions live on, but individuals die—and with them much of their experience and knowledge. We teach people who live a handful of decades and then die, their education gone forever. If we are lucky, they have passed on what they could; their teaching becomes the seeds for the next generation. We are like gardeners concentrating solely on annuals that bloom brightly but need replanting every spring. Living longer, we may no longer squander education, but rather invest in perennials that bloom for many more years. Education will have more value as the return extends over a hundred or more years instead of a few decades. Elementary education will diminish as a part of the economy, as the very young become a smaller percentage of the population, but, as an investment in our lives, training and education will be more important than ever.

The arts, especially the entertainment industry, should flourish, with the greater demand from those at leisure and the disposable income to support them. Retaining older artists should result in greater mastery, but coupled with greater conservatism. In the arts and sciences, the novel does not triumph so much by greater mastery as by lesser mortality. The old will remain—perhaps a thorn in the side of the young—and the young will have to put up with them.

Medicine will be affected in the same way as the arts, the sciences, and education, but in one additional way: Much of our current medicine will become superfluous, though new techniques will take its place. The defining mark of any profession is that it works to make itself unnecessary. In this, medicine soon will have unprecedented success. Currently, one seventh of the gross national product of the United States is spent on health care. In most cases, telomere therapy will cut medical costs. Hospitals will change their focus, concentrating on infections, trauma, psychiatric intervention, and genetic diseases rather than the diseases of aging. The nursing home industry will show the most dramatic change, but there will be time to adapt. Those patients already in nursing homes will likely remain; they may even stay longer as telomere therapy makes many of them healthier but no less dependent. These will be the chronic patients, while in the decades to come, new patients will become progressively rarer. Over the next two decades, hospitals will have time to adjust both their training of new staff and their capital investments to match the changing patient population.

Individual specialties will be affected in different ways. Most of a cardiologist's practice now involves treating the diseases caused by aging vessels, and will largely disappear. Those specialties dependent on the diseases we associate with aging will find themselves with a narrowing and healthier patient base. Others, such as general surgeons, pediatricians, obstetricians, and psychiatrists, will be relatively unaffected. Oncologists won't be out of business, but their practice will shift dramatically away from long-term battles against a recurring enemy and toward detection and rapid, inexpensive, and painless cures.

Will all medical costs be lowered? If demand for other medical care increases at the same time, there might be no decrease in net costs. Suppose, for example, that the cost of services falls 50 percent owing to telomere therapy, but at the same time we demand that our insurers, or the government, underwrite full dental care, sports therapy, genetic testing, genetic alteration, psychiatric care, nutritional counseling, and therapeutic vacations. Although the cost of *current services* would fall, the net cost—and so our health insurance premiums or Medicare taxes—would rise if we demand more medical care.

And what will happen in a century? Medical costs are likely to fall drastically for a time but will then return. Disease, like death, will never be conquered completely, nor will medical costs. How high these deferred costs are will depend on what diseases occur. Curing many childhood illnesses only postponed the medical costs until those same children grew old enough to have the heart attacks and cancers that we now die of at far greater expense. Future cost may remain low. We will live longer, spreading out the cost of disease over a much longer lifetime and giving us more time to save and pay for it. If every twenty-five-year-old had a heart attack, we would have only a few years, subtracting childhood and the employment training period, to earn the money to pay the medical bills. But if we live three times that long, we spread out the cost over a longer employment life. And if we double our life spans, we will have a longer life and a much longer earning period in which to balance any cost increase. Over the next few centuries, medical costs may remain low, compared with our capacity to pay for them, without any financially significant rebound.

What will happen to stocks and bonds? A large percentage of the population have their money invested in the market, especially in pension funds.[25] As we live longer, our investments will increase. As more people invest in equities, and the demand goes up, prices will rise—and subsequent returns may eventually decrease. If I work for forty years and retire for twenty, I require a certain return on my pension. But if I work for eighty years, I don't need as much return to retire for twenty years. Portfolios will emphasize long-term gains. Investment capital, and with it venture capital, will make more money available for start-up companies, industrial expansion, and research.

The overall outlook for the economy is excellent. Although there are negative features to the future economy—urban sprawl, pollution, heavier highway use, higher land costs, etc.—most of these will not be made any worse because we live longer. One ironic outcome is that we will no longer be as able to pass on the national debt to our children; it will still be ours as well as theirs.

THE SOCIAL WEAVE

The older I grow, the more I distrust the familiar doctrine that age brings wisdom.

—H. L. MENCKEN

The worth of any advance can best be measured in social units. But the measure should not be how many houses we can build or how many jobs we have created, but whether we are better people for having done so. How many of us are truly happy; in other words, how well do we treat one another.

What will happen to us when we extend our lives? We have considered the question from several perspectives. We have looked at medicine, predicting what we could cure and what we could not. We have tried to predict what would happen to our jobs and to our economy. How else will we change if we live longer, healthier lives? What will become of our parents, our brothers, our sisters, our spouses, and our children? What about our friends? These are more important questions.

CRIME AND VIOLENCE

Most violent crimes are committed by those younger than forty years of age. Perhaps it is because we gain in wisdom as we age, or perhaps because we simply grow too tired and too old for violence. Violence may be a matter of getting used to our young bodies, our lives, our world. As we live longer, the average age of the population will shift upward and with it our average behavior. The tenor of our civilization will shift. A portion of this will be self-selection. Those engaging in violent activities die young because they antagonize others. Whatever the selection pressure, whether it is Darwinian or simply a matter of getting old enough to know better, the middle-aged are seldom violent compared with their juniors, and it is on this observation we might best pin our hopes. The world should slowly, but quite literally, grow up.

THE WORLD

Telomere therapy cannot cure dysentery, starvation, and land mine injuries. The poorer areas of our world have far deeper problems than telomere shortening. The leading cause of death in Egypt is dysentery, not vessel disease; in Mexico, it is accidents, not cancer; in the Philippines, pneumonia and influenza, not strokes.[26] Although telomere therapy is likely to alter the life span of those who would otherwise die of vessel diseases and cancer, it has very little to offer those whose water supply is contaminated. All of the telomeres in the world cannot replace a clean well or a peace agreement.

Much of the medical care in developed countries prolongs the lives of those of us with no future and who can no longer recall their past, who have no hope and no wish to remain alive. Yearly we spend billions for little return, purchasing a few more weeks, or days, or hours, for a life that has already past. Telomere therapy breaks from this practice, promising us healthy lives that can contribute to others, even those who need only a new well.

Abraham Lincoln remarked that you can't help a weak man by destroying the life of a strong one. Nor do you save a life in Rwanda by letting someone die in New York. *You save lives by saving lives;* the location is immaterial. The question is what you save them for, not where they live. If we save people from the diseases of the old, perhaps they in turn can save others from the diseases of the young.

SOCIAL ROLES

We have usually expected our elders to behave differently from our children. Children were expected to behave in a more irresponsible fashion than adults. Age roles may grow more complex; we may see those over a hundred shunning "youngsters" of ninety, much as some retirement communities currently forbid families with young children. Older people, still healthy and independent with a long employment history, will be well off financially, well connected politically, and savvy about defending their perquisites and their social role from the young and still disenfranchised.

But it may be difficult to tell who is old and who is young. Up until now, distinct age roles have been supported by visible differences. The visible differences will largely disappear. As we become less certain of someone else's age, age roles become less enforceable.

If we go back a thousand years, anyone making it to age forty was not only old, but experienced—and therefore commanded respect. Most died young either from infection or accidents. The "elderly" were likely to be physically active and independent or they were dead. It was natural to respect elders.

Presently, anyone who makes it to eighty is experienced, but we think of them as dependent. The majority of eighty-year-olds are healthy, but there is little respect for age. We associate age with what we fear rather than what we respect.

Telomere therapy may give us new cause to respect age. Anyone who makes it to a century and a half will be experienced—not "aged." They will be independent—not disabled—and they will still be respected. We are likely to again come to emulate the old: They will have been successful, will be healthy, and will be far more knowledgeable than the young. They are also more likely to be in charge. Respect for the elderly will have come full circle.

There will also probably exist prejudice against those who do not receive treatments and who therefore "look old," but the more likely prejudice will be against the young. Prejudice will survive, but can age prejudice remain when we cannot tell the difference in years? We may base our prejudices on what people know and what they have so far achieved, relying upon indications of wealth, success, or fashion.

How will telomere therapy affect sexual roles? Biologists would point out that a large portion of the role difference has been attributable to the different requirements concerning having and raising children: A woman had to invest a minimum of nine months in pregnancy; a man only required a few minutes. In most societies, however, both sexes were expected to spend as long as another two decades raising their mutual children. Twenty years is a long time, particularly if your average life span was only twenty-five.

This aspect of life is proportionately much less now than ever before. It may take twenty years to raise a child, but if a woman lives for seventy-five, what is her role afterward? If a man is to provide for children for the same time period, what is his role afterward? The number of years that remain to us after raising children has been growing steadily and is about to grow enormously as telomere therapy becomes available. There will be all the less support for distinct social sex roles as our lives extend into a century or more.

This assumes that menopause will not be postponed by telomere therapy. Female fertility would still end halfway through the first century, without adding any further impetus to reinforcement of distinct sex roles—as it would if menopause is also postponed by telomere therapy. If menopause is unchanged, the economic, legal, and social distinctions between sex roles will grow less discernible as we live longer lives, women and men will become even more similar in terms of their earnings, their status, and their social functions. It is not that we will become sexless, androgynous creatures: far from it. We can expect that anatomic differences will be maintained even more clearly than they are now and that sexual activities will be all the more common when people are healthy and active.

And what about men? They will almost certainly remain fertile for a longer period, which will maintain some support for sex role distinctions: A man will probably still be able to be a parent at 150, a woman probably won't. But having children has a much greater impact on a woman's professional and social life than it has on a man's. It is this difference that will begin to decrease if menopause is unaffected. Perhaps it will be the older woman who is freer to pursue a career, while a man's career will suffer from being in the "daddy track" if he wants to be a father at 150, an ironic reversal if it occurs.

SOCIAL INSTITUTIONS

The institutions of family and marriage are all but universal. Neither one is strictly and independently a social institution: Both have biological roots and biological constraints. How will these institutions change because we live longer? Families may become multigenerational[27] and therefore larger, but they are not likely to live under one roof. The historical trend is clearly toward smaller families. Nuclear families (living under the same roof) rarely encompass three generations anymore and even when they include only two generations it is usually limited to the two decades it takes to raise children. In an increasing number of cases, the nuclear family unit is now limited to a child and a single parent. Such families have increased markedly since 1960, and more than a third of all children now live with a parent who has never been married at all.[28] If the trend continues, never-married parents—never mind the divorced one—will be in the majority by the end of this century. How will a longer life span affect the trend?

Dual careers have already put a strain on marriages. When one spouse has a job in London and the other is offered an excellent prospect in New York, it puts great pressure on the marriage. Longer life will only add to this trend; as the opportunities to change careers multiply, so will the chances of marriages failing. It is unlikely that one partner will be without a career for a century of marriage after raising children. The divorce rate will continue climbing and so will the never-married parenting rate.

Nor is that the only reason that marriages will continue declining. Some marriages are maintained simply by the fear of dying alone, the couples considering divorce unacceptable simply because they need a hand to hold in the face of their onrushing mortality. But if they know they can be healthy for another fifty years, they may not tolerate a spouse they have grown apart from. Of course, some marriages among the elderly are the more solid for the years spent building them and will remain, not only in sickness but in health.

Nuclear families that live together will continue to shrink. However, the prediction for the *extended family*—defined as all your relatives—is vastly different. Already as our lives have grown longer, there are more families whose collection of living grandparents, in-laws, ex-spouses, stepparents, and various other relatives are growing year by year. This extended family will grow enormously larger: We may have family get-togethers where great-great-great-great-grandparents happily play with the youngest children, where much of the initial social conversation focuses on trying to remember the relationship between you and the person you just met again for the first time in fifty years.

The generation gap will probably become smaller. Not only will it be more difficult to tell old from young, but their activities will overlap more. You may be skating with your great-grandmother when she is ninety-five. The old have, until now, been less likely to indulge in the activities of the young, but we will surely see more centenarians using in-line skates, scuba diving, and doing gymnastics than we currently do. As the difference in physical activities breaks down, so to some degree may the generation gap.

However, the generation gap is also the expression of differences in experience and maturity. An eighteen-year-old is willing to take risks that few of us would take at thirty, let alone sixty. How many bungee jumpers will there be who are ninety—though every bit as physically fit as a thirty-year-old? And how many race car drivers, technical mountain climbers, hand gliders, and parachute jumpers?

LEGAL CHANGES

Telomere therapy may cause several changes in the law. To the extent that it is seen as contributing to population growth, it may increase the likelihood of laws that restrict fertility. Whether that is good or bad—or both—the social pressures for such laws and the odds of them passing will increase as the world's population does. What about voting rights? Currently most countries restrict voting to those older than about two decades, the exact age depending on the country, local government options, and the kind of election. We might see this age limit raised as we disenfranchise the "young"—perhaps those under fifty?

"Life" prison terms will be another problem. Should "life" mean until you reach 75 or until you die, even if that takes two centuries? Will the sentence include free telomere treatment as part of the prison medical care or specifically exclude it? Will twenty years in prison, when people will live to 150, be comparable with ten years served today, when we only live to 75? Most European countries mete out few sentences greater than about a decade and a half: Murder is typically punished by a seven- to fifteen-year sentence. Even where the sentence is indeterminate—"at Her Majesty's pleasure" in England—the end result usually averages the same number of years. This is unlikely to change in Europe; it is likely that the American system of sentencing will change, mainly because as our life spans increase, so will the cost to taxpayers of a life sentence. We will opt either for the death penalty or for sentences shorter than life. But the trend is away from capital punishment: Each year, on the average, two more countries abolish it.[29]

Although most developed nations have abolished the death penalty, the prominent exception is the United States. Even in the United States, the judicial trend (in the Supreme Court, for example) has been to restrict the death penalty. Public opinion, and consequently legislative opinion, changes with the year and with crime statistics, but the long-term trend is also away from the death penalty in the United States.

More important than what those not in prison will think about sentences is what prisoners themselves will feel. When ten years is one fifth of one's adult life and one is middle-aged, will ten years be enough of a deterrent to prevent most crimes? Telomere therapy may change sentencing, but there is no clear way to predict how it will do so.

THE INDIVIDUAL

The youth gets together his materials to build a bridge to the moon, or, perchance, a palace or temple on the earth, and, at length, the middle-aged man concludes to build a woodshed with them.

—Henry David Thoreau, *Walden*

We did not go to the moon to collect minerals. We did not even go because it was good science or a demonstration of technical prowess; we went because we had dreamed of it for thousands of years. Conquering aging will give us more than years and cures for disease; it will give us our dreams. Longevity therapy renews those dreams: The limits of life become unknown and—to an extent not previously true—determined by ourselves and what we do with our bodies and our souls.

What will telomere therapy do to our capabilities? What if Albert Einstein were still active and young, perhaps working hard on superstring theory? What if Martha Graham were still directing her own dance pieces, and as capable of dancing them as she was at thirty? What if Claude Monet were still painting in Giverney? What if Mozart hadn't died at thirty-five, but had composed for another century?

But what if creative minds are less creative? Subrahmanyan Chandrasekhar, one of the most creative astrophysicists of our century, was once asked such a question. How could someone who had been so consistently productive simply stop working after he finished writing his book on the life of Sir Isaac Newton? "Obviously I can go on doing work of a quality that is below my standards, but why do that?" he replied. "So the time must come when I say, 'Stop.' "[30] If we grow stale, we will stop ourselves. If we don't, others will surpass us. As a society, we will not lose in the process.

And what of our responsibilities? As we grow older, we have more responsibility for others and for ourselves. We acquire children, family, homes, all of which—emotionally, physically, or financially—depend on us. We grow up and learn that, to a remarkable degree, our lives are a product of our own actions. This will be even more true when we remove the afflictions of aging. Aging doesn't care who you are or what you have accomplished; you still grow old. But if we can reverse aging, then what happens to us will be determined—to a far greater degree than ever before—by our own actions.

Much of this increase in personal responsibility will involve self-selection. Those who won't take responsibility for their health won't survive; we will be forced to become wise. Of course, this is not an absolute; there will always be old fools, just as there are wise youngsters. On the average, however, the paradigm that age brings greater wisdom is accurate: There are relatively few frivolous, impatient, foolish old people.

Longer life, shorn of the diseases of aging, promises us a windfall in wisdom. We are likely to be more responsible and to take more responsibility.

RELIGION AND ETHICS

On a bridge suspended over a precipice
Clings an ivy vine, body and soul together.

—BASHO, "A VISIT TO SARASHIMA VILLAGE"

RELIGION

Once, when I was visiting a Tibetan monastery, two Thai monks asked me to clarify the differences between "a few minor sects in Western religion." Wondering how much I really could remember about the differences among Methodists, Baptists, Seventh Day Adventists, Mormons, Episcopalians, Catholics, and dozens more, I asked which sects had them confused. Their "minor sects" were Judaism, Christianity, and Islam.

About one third of the world's population is Christian; about one sixth, Muslim; one eighth, Hindu; one twentieth, Buddhist; and about one in three hundred is Jewish. In the United States, about 90 percent of us are Christian (half Protestants, almost that many Catholics, and a small number of Eastern Orthodox), about 2 percent of us are Jews, and roughly the same percentage are Muslims.[31]

What will these religions have to say about extending the human life span? Consider the Judeo-Christian perspective. Will religious leaders accept the offer of a longer health span? Will they give religious reasons for doing so, or not doing so? Francis Schaeffer, who was the leader of L'Abri, a think tank for the evangelical Protestant community, was once asked," "If there were a pill that when taken reversed the aging process and prevented subsequent aging, would you take it?" His response was illuminating: "Yes, because the aging process is a consequence of the historic fall of man and it is our duty as Christians—inasmuch as it is in our power—to undo the work of the fall."[32]

When we halt aging, are we interfering with the will of God or, as Francis Schaeffer suggests, following his commands all the more closely? Is it interference to cure cancer or does God intend that we do so? Is it interference to prevent heart disease or God's will that patients suffer? And is it interference to try to give children back their childhood and adults back their lives? The answer is clear to those of us who have spent our lives trying to cure others.

Jesus raised Lazarus from the dead. Can a long and healthy life be an affront to God?

> *I have come that men may have life and may have it in all its fullness.* [John 10:10]

In John 9, Jesus was criticized for healing on the Sabbath, when he gave sight to a man blind since birth. But others asked:

> *How could such signs come from a sinner?* [John 9:16]

How indeed? Healing is no sin. Jesus healed, he brought life, he opened our eyes.

In Christian teaching, there is a clear emphasis on the quality of life.

Righteousness is not a question of length of life, but of living a good, spiritual life. As we live today, we age and die. Treated with telomere therapy, we will still age and die, but we will live much longer. Can it be immoral to decline treatment? Certainly not. How could it be any more immoral to decline telomere therapy than to do so for cancer therapy, surgery, or antibiotics? Declining these therapies may be foolish, stubborn, or fatal, but it is not a sin, nor would it be a sin to decline therapy aimed at a longer, healthier life.

Does God intend that we limit our lives? Death cannot be evaded, but does God give us a specific limit? In Genesis 6:3, God says:

> *My spirit shall not always strive in me for the sake*
> *of man, for that he is but flesh; and his days shall*
> *be a hundred and twenty years.*

Is this then a limit? It is biologically. The maximum human life span is about 120. Has God said that this is it, we cannot have any more, or that this is all he helps us with and that beyond that we must work for it? The Hebrew word in this verse is ידון (pronounced Y'don), meaning to strive, remain, or abide. It is used in the sense of to abide within God: God will abide with us for these years. He did not say that we were not to strive, or that we must have no more years, or that he would desert us; only that this much was his gift.

Do we have a right to a longer life? The idea of a right to anything—life or health, for example—is a new one; nowhere is it present in the Bible. Rabbi Lord I. Jakobovits, a biblical scholar and ethicist, points out that nowhere in the Old Testament—or anywhere in classical Hebrew for that matter—is there even a word for "rights."[33] Rather there are *mitzvot:* obligations, duties, and commandments. God gives commandments, not rights. The most important commandment is to keep the Sabbath, yet even this one is overridden by the duty to save a life. We lack a right to life; we have a duty to life. Our duty is to maintain life, a life that is infinite in value, whether it lasts hours, days, years, or centuries. Life is no more valuable for lasting twice as long—and no less valuable, either. While we have no right to a longer life, we have a *duty* to protect the life we have, however long it may be, however long it may become.

Telomere therapy extends life and is therefore a good from the rabbinical standpoint. The same could be said of preventing the diseases of aging: Not only do we meet the commandment to preserve life, but we prevent suffering as well. Rabbi J. David Bleich wrote on the medical ethics of genetic engineering:

> *Because we regard healing as an obligation, not as an option, we are obliged to preserve life. We are obliged to preserve our own life, and we are obliged to preserve someone else's life when we can.*[34]

It is morally imperative, within the Jewish ethical tradition, to perfect a therapy that could save lives. The underlying duty grows from the possibility that health and long life may give us a better chance to obey God and fulfill our duties. An ability to save lives makes it imperative that we do so.[35]

Will life be improved by simply being longer? Perhaps we will be wiser or more compassionate for having lived longer. Job, having lived a life that was as long as it was difficult, asked the same question, a question that suggests his answer:

> *Is not wisdom found among the aged? Does not long life bring understanding?* [Job 12:12]

As we age, do we have the same duty to gain wisdom that we have to cherish life? Yes; we have a duty to learn and to grow; added years only add to our duty. In the Judeo-Christian tradition, age gives us the chance to improve and the responsibility to do so.

Islamic ethics strongly reflect the same tradition: We live mainly to do good, and beyond that our lives have little meaning. The length of our life should be determined by how much good we can do. We see this in the traditional Islamic prayer from *Sahifa al-Sajjadiyya:*

O my Lord, make my life long in order for me
to do all the good; and make it short in order
to protect me from committing evil.[36]

The prospect of a long life is itself neither good nor bad; it is a chance to do good or it is nothing.

The prophet Noah, for instance, lived 950 years. He "found favor in the eyes of the Lord" (Genesis 6:5), because he preached the word of God. He was saved because he was a believing man (Koran, Sura 51:28, Nu). He gave warning to the people, even though they continued to "thrust their fingers in their ears" and "magnify themselves in pride" (Sura 51:7, Nu). God can "bend us backward" (Sura 36:68), restoring youth and giving us long life if we are worthy.

In each of the three religions that make up the Western heritage—Judaism, Christianity, and Islam—God sets the span of our lives, but it is the morality of our actions that determines the worth of our lives.

The two major Eastern religions—Hinduism and Buddhism—might be expected to have less interest in the question of extending the life span. In both of these religions contain the concept of rebirth, providing us with several lifetimes, so there would seem to be little need to extend a single lifetime out of those many.

Yet there exists a substantial religious literature—particularly within Hinduism—that supports the extension of life span and rejuvenation. The best example is in the Ayurvedic literature (Ayurvedic literally means "signs of long life." In the *Carakasamhita*, for instance, priests go to the physician of the gods and ask how they may extend life.[37] The physician's response makes up most of the first volume. The second volume deals specifically with extending life by the use of medicines. Although many early Hindu texts view normal life as being a century long, there is a long tradition of texts on life extension, including the Bower Texts from the early fourth century, which describe exactly what medications and chemicals will extend life beyond the classical century.

More interesting than the techniques is the rationale for a long, healthy life. The gods explain that we should try to stay healthy as long as possible because disease and early death interfere with our religious obligations.[38] In Hinduism, as in Judaism, health is not only desirable to avoid suffering for its own sake but, more important, it is a way to meet our obligations to God. Good health allows us to follow God's commandments. In the Hindu tradition, seeking and maintaining your health is a religious duty.

In Buddhism, as in Hinduism, there is a traditional interest in rejuvenation—in part borrowed from Taoism, in part perhaps from the earlier Hindu soil from which Buddhism sprang. For the majority of mainstream Buddhists, the length of life is less of a religious issue than it is a personal one. The emphasis is on attainment of nirvana, but still—as in Western traditions—the question is not so much how long your life is (or your lives have been) as how worthy it is. Do you follow the correct—in this case the eightfold—path to enlightenment?

More to the point in Buddhism is the issue of "attachment." In the Buddhist view, all suffering derives from your attachment to things or beliefs. If you are no longer attached to things in the world, then you won't suffer when you lose them. This is especially true of life itself. Life and death are a unity. As the Reverend Daishin Morgan, abbot of a Buddhist monastery, says:

> Our notion of sacredness becomes confused with a duality of thinking that life is good and death is bad. We can never find peace within this split. Once the realistic possibility of longevity treatment exists, the prospect of wise reflection having much impact on the impatient grasping of it as another "fundamental human right" seems remote.[39]

The Buddhist concern is that we may become so foolishly attached to life—all the more so if we have the chance to extend it—that we forget the deeper, more important issues: suffering and freeing ourselves from attachment. Those should be the primary concern, not life. We are here to escape suffering, not death. The Western religions value life itself and stress the importance of a moral life; in Buddhism the very act of clinging to life prevents it from being moral. Life—no matter how far we extend it—is no more to be sought after than is death; what matters more is freedom from either. We should rise above life, death, and suffering; seek understanding rather than longer life. Long life is irrelevant to following the path of the Buddha.[40]

Throughout the world, in perhaps all religions, we are driven back to the same consideration: not how long life can be maintained, not even the quality of life, but the quality of the person who lives it. It matters little, from the perspective of religion, when you died or how you suffered; it matters a great deal *how* you lived. God was perfectly willing to test Job by destroying his family, his property, and his health. Job suffered, but Job remained devout. In Buddhism, the assumption is that all life—yours as well as Job's—is suffering. But the question is, do you follow the higher path, not, have you suffered.

In each religion, it matters little how long life lasts, but it matters very much what you do with that life. This perspective is no recommendation for a short life, rife with disease. To the contrary, a long life and good health provide a greater opportunity to do good and to live a moral life. We are not given grace, but a chance to earn it.

ETHICAL ASPECTS

The difference between a moral man and a man of honor is that the latter regrets a discreditable act, even when it has worked and he has not been caught.

—H. L. MENCKEN

Every scientific advance brings ethical questions. Such advances are not intrinsically unethical, but they bring novel opportunities to behave unethically. Nor are advances inherently ethical—although they offer opportunities for ethical behavior.

Telomere therapy offers most to those who survive long enough to grow old. The Third World has little time to waste with the current issues that rack Western medical ethics. There are more basic issues: dehydration, fever, malnutrition. The evil is clear, ethical questions few. The question of whether to resuscitate an elderly person with multiple diseases and an uncertain mental status is common in the hospitals of developed countries; it is hypothetical in much of the world, a question that the Third World wishes it had the luxury to ask.

Developed—affluent—countries worry about the quality of life and the timing of death; about stroke, cancer, and heart disease. The concerns of poorer countries are food, water, and shelter; plague, famine, and war. The developed countries worry about medical ethics; the undeveloped countries worry about having any medical care at all—they are "without adequate and decent health services ... which may be the real ethical crisis."[41]

The Judeo-Christian tradition, and that of many other religions, is correct: All lives are equal. The ethical perspective is no different: All lives are equally valuable. Even though we don't harm anyone in Somalia by saving a life in Ohio, we do *spiritual* damage if we *only* save lives in Ohio and consider them more valuable than those in Somalia. They are not. Nor are they more valuable in Somalia. We must save lives where we are able to.

The fact that others suffer en masse elsewhere does not absolve us from making ethical decisions in our daily lives. We will be faced with our own—necessarily personal, local, and individual—ethical problems whether we work diligently to help others or not, whether we succeed in helping or not, whether we are even aware of the suffering of others or not.

We already wrestle with ethical dilemmas (e.g., resuscitation with little chance of survival), but telomere therapy gives them new holds. The first ethical issue is whether or not we—or those we love—should take it. The answer seems clear at first: Yes, because in doing so, aren't we trying to prevent or reverse disease and suffering? Telomere therapy offers health and longer life without disease. So it seems every bit as simple an issue as whether or not to give an antibiotic for an infection or to cure a child of leukemia.

Yet do we give antibiotics to the elderly patient with terminal cancer, Alzheimer's disease, and a pneumonia who is dependent on a respirator? Do we give a final treatment of chemotherapy—knowing there is little chance of success—to the child who, sick and frightened, begs us not to? Perhaps not, and the answer applies to telomere therapy as well.

Like antibiotics and vaccinations, telomere therapy offers health and a moderate guarantee against disease, but not without presenting difficult ethical questions. There is an elderly man, the patient of a physician I know, who is frail, but still healthy. He has been married to the same woman for fifty-five years. His wife has Alzheimer's and, on bad days, doesn't recognize him. Even on good days she can't remember his name. Her husband loves her, cares for her, is devoted to her. Left alone, she will be dead in a few years. His only wish is that he will live long enough to tuck her in one final time and, soon afterward, die himself.

What if we can offer both of them health and longer lives? We could, perhaps, make him twenty again, active and vigorous, far more able to care for her. We could, perhaps, make her younger as well, and certainly healthier in most ways. But we cannot give her back her mind; we cannot cure her Alzheimer's.

In his place, what would you do? Would you opt for telomere treatment for yourself alone, knowing you could better care for her? You might be able to keep her more comfortable and lessen the chance that she would be left alone by your death. Or would you remain frail and hope for the best? Or treat her, too, knowing that she would be young again but not whole?

Physicians are asked to "do everything they can" for someone who is *already* gone: biologically alive perhaps, but in all other ways long gone, with only the family holding them back. What will happen to these patients? Will the family demand that they be treated, brought back to useless youth and maintained for another lifetime with pain, dementia, and failed organs?

If my mind is gone, will my family understand that my previous wishes—that I should not be given longevity treatment—are to be respected? Will the physicians? Will the courts? Most families, most physicians, and most courts today *do* respect such wishes. The possibility of longevity therapy adds a twist, however. There is currently little to gain—even for bereft family members—by extending the life a few uncertain hours, days, or weeks. The delay gives them time to ease into mourning, little else. If we can turn back aging, however, we might offer years more. How could a family not be tempted? And what physician will be sure that, in years to come, more cannot be done? These are painful decisions: We are asked to let someone we love die, perhaps knowing it is the right decision, but wishing to the bottom of our souls that it was not. Death is final and hope strong.

How will we deal with changes in resuscitation? When will we be aggressive and when quiet in the face of death? Most physicians are more aggressive in trying to resuscitate children than adults. Children have more to live for and are more likely to survive our attempts to retrieve them. Suddenly, all of this will change. Should we give the seventy-year-old the same chance we give the child of seven? Will our aggressive efforts carry over into every case?

Even to consider these ethical issues is our fortune. We worry about whether we should resuscitate the ninety-year-old with terminal cancer. What father of a starving four-year-old wouldn't give his own life to let his child live to be five, let alone live to be ninety—cancer or not? Many people in this world envy our dilemmas. We have inherited ethical problems as a trivial cost of our immense fortune. And soon, we will have new ethical problems as our lives grow longer and healthier. The questions will alter, but we will still be faced with the underlying question not of death versus life, but of how we die—and why we live.

WERE YOU TO LIVE...

Were you to live three thousand years, or even thirty thousand, remember that the sole life which a man can lose is that which he is living at the moment ... the longest life and the shortest amount to the same thing.

—MARCUS AURELIUS, *MEDITATIONS*, *BOOK TWO*

Life is not merely a matter of years. It is a quality. Faced with a choice between living fifty years with Alzheimer's disease and five years with robust health followed by sudden death, which would you choose? Although you may live for centuries, it matters little if you have not lived well. What is it that makes a life worthwhile?

Living for a century does not of itself deserve respect; it gives you the opportunity to earn it. Your life will be judged by the character you display and the effect you have on the lives of others. What will you do if you live for a century? If you are given two, will you accomplish more? A longer life should be held to a higher standard. There is no fault in dying young and friendless, but no defense for living long without them. Living a long, healthy life is an opportunity that few now have. But with long life comes an obligation to ourselves and to those we share our lives with.

Our lives are given, but they are also made. You create your life day by day, and only you can make your life better. Were we to cure all disease and enable you to live forever, it would not make you one whit nobler than you are now. That will not happen unless you make it so. Your life, and the lives of those around you, are about to change. The change will be for the better if you make it so. What you will do with that change, and with the longer life it creates for you, will ultimately have little to do with your telomeres, or your cells, or your life span, and nothing to do with this book. It will have everything to do with you. May your life be long, healthy, and well lived.

G L O S S A R Y

apoptosis—programmed cell death, or cell "suicide," occurring at the instruction (signal) of neighboring cells or of hormones from more distant cells. See *necrosis*.

bystander cell—a cell that is adversely affected by a process occurring in another cell

catalase (CAT)—a protective enzyme responsible for metabolizing free radicals. See also *SOD*.

chromosome—a long, chained molecule in which are written the genes; usually linear, but occasionally circular

DDBPs (damaged DNA binding proteins)—protein monitors that prevent cells from passing on genetic errors

DHEA (dehydroepiandrosterone)—the most common steroid in the blood, whose levels decline with age

DNA (deoxyribonucleic acid)—a family of molecules that make up the double helix strands that are the basis of heredity and cell replication

DNA polymerase—any of several enzymes that replicate or repair DNA; "Xerox machines" of the genetic realm, responsible for replicating the chromosome

double helix—the form of a DNA chromosome, a spiral made of two strands held together by cross-links

entropy—the tendency of all systems to disintegrate; the forces of disintegration, decay, and chaos

enzymes—substances produced by living cells that act as catalysts for molecular reactions within the body

euchromatin—that portion of a chromosome that is unwound and available for use by the cell

eukaryote—an organism having one or more cells with nuclei

fibroblast—a cell that produces connective tissue

free radical—a molecule with a single unpaired electron in its outermost shell, which "steals" an electron from another molecule, causing damage in doing so

germ cell—an egg or sperm cell, set apart from the rest of the body to unite with a cell of the opposite sex to form a new organism. See *somatic cell*.

Hayflick limit—the limit on the number of generations over which a cell may divide. There is a different Hayflick limit for each different kind of cell.

HeLa cell—an ovarian cancer cell used in biomedical research

heterochromatin—the portion of a chromosome that remains tightly wound and unavailable. See *euchromatin*.

homeostasis—a tendency toward the maintenance of stable systems within the body

Humpty-Dumpty effect—loss of cells that cannot be replaced, resulting from various diseases

Hutchinson-Gilford syndrome—a rare progeric disease in which children typically die by age thirteen, having acquired the physical features of old age. See *Werner's syndrome*.

kilobase—unit of measurement of DNA strands; a thousand bases

leukocyte—a white blood cell important to immune function

lipofuscin—a brown pigment similar to melanin, found in certain older tissues that have degenerated into exhaustion

melatonin—a hormone secreted by the pineal gland, whose levels decline with aging

necrosis—the most frequent kind of cell death, caused by an inadequate environment. See *apoptosis*.

SOD (superoxide dismutase)—a protective enzyme responsible for metabolizing free radicals. See also *catalase*.

somatic cell—one of the cells that become differentiated and make up the body's individual tissues and organs; distinguished from a *germ cell*

stem cell—a relatively undifferentiated, usually embryonic cell existing in the bone marrow that produces other more differentiated cells

telomerase—an enzyme, part protein and part RNA, that extends the telomere. See *telomere*.

telomerase inducer—a substance introduced into a cell to stimulate the production of telomerase. See *telomerase inhibitor*.

telomerase inhibitor—a substance introduced into a cell to prevent telomerase function. See *telomerase inducer*.

telomere—one of the ends of each of the four "arms" of a chromosome

telomere therapy—treatment of chromosomes to lengthen their telomeres in order to prevent further aging of the cells to which they belong, for the ultimate purpose of increasing the human life span. In the case of cancer cells, treatment of the cells in order to prevent telomerase function and destroy the cells

trophic factors—local hormones that control the functions and division of other cells

Werner's syndrome—a progeric disease typically presenting in the twenties and causing apparent premature aging and death by age fifty. See *Hutchinson-Gilford syndrome*.

N O T E S

Chapter 1: Life

1. On the other hand, the distinction is occasionally cloudy and the issue of aging at all an uncertain one in certain invertebrate species. See Rose's excellent review, 1991, p. 84ff. This issue is irrelevant, to invertebrates in general and humans in particular, to this discussion. Rose himself, always brilliant and prudent, finally comes down in favor of the universality of aging in somatic, as opposed to germ, cells in species in which the distinction can be made (p. 90).
2. Beck, 1983.
3. SOD, or superoxide dismutase, is actually a family of proteins. The best evidence that it is critical to aging is probably that of Orr and Sohal, 1994.

Chapter 2: The Engines of Aging

1. This is generally true, but like everything in biology, there are exceptions. See Kreil, 1994.
2. More precisely, the amino acids making up proteins all twist to the left, but sugar molecules—including those attached to DNA and RNA molecules—all twist to the right. Why they do so is a fascinating question, but beyond the scope of our discussion. See Cohen, 1995.
3. Stern, 1993.
4. 23 kilocalories.
5. Or others such as superoxide, hydroxyl, lipid peroxide, alkoxyl, and peroxyl radicals.
6. Yu, 1993, p. 60.
7. Ibid. p. 75 and Chapter 5.
8. Such as histidine, lysine, proline, and arginine.
9. Floyd, 1993.
10. More than 10^{21}.

11. Thymine and cytosine.
12. Cells of the inferior olive, for example.
13. Meites, Hylka, and Sonntag, 1984, p. 195.
14. See, for example, Orgel, 1963, 1973.
15. Amenta, 1993; Arking, 1991, Chapter 5.
16. Singer and Berg, 1991, p. 107.
17. Singer and Berg, 1991.
18. Harley, 1988.
19. Matsuo, 1993, p. 145; Yu, 1993.
20. Arking, 1991, p. 307.
21. Fraga et al., 1990.
22. Or in the microsomes.
23. Tan et al., 1993.
24. Matsuo, 1993; Yu, 1993.
25. Yu, 1993, pp. 71–72.
26. Yu, 1993, p. 72.
27. Weindruch et al., 1993.
28. It is interesting to note that antioxidant enzymes may even increase with age, at least in muscles. Luhtala et al., 1994.
29. Stern, 1993.
30. Conley, 1974.
31. Fefer, 1977.
32. Arking, 1991, p. 326.
33. If the damage rate is constant at 1%, the total number of plants is 100, the number taken out every day (t) varies (but is equal to the number put back in), and the number of damaged plants at any time is X, then if the number of damaged plants on any given day is X_N, the next day the number of damaged plants will be X_{N+1}. So the formula for each day is the damage rate (1), plus the number remaining damaged from the previous day (X_N), minus the percentage of previously damaged plants likely to be removed by turnover ($\frac{tX_N}{100}$):

$$X_{N+1} = 1 + (X_N) - [(X_N)(\frac{t}{100})]$$

When the system comes to equilibrium X_N will equal X_{N+1}. So:

$$X = 1 + \frac{X\,(100-t)}{100}$$

When the turnover rate is 50%:

$$X = 1 + .5X$$
$$= 2$$

When the turnover rate is 2%:

$$X = 1 + .98\,X$$
$$= 50$$

34. Yu, 1993, p. 46
35. Yu, 1993 pp. 74, 143ff., 149. On the other hand, see Luhtala et al., 1994.
36. Yu, 1993, pp. 69–70,
37. Ibid. pp. 69–70, 74.
38. Luhtala et al., 1994, would apparently disagree, at least in their animal model.
39. And microsomes.
40. Yu, 1993, p. 60.
41. Ibid. p. 65ff.
42. Ibid. p. 78ff.
43. Ibid, p. 58.
44. Heinlein, 1958.
45. Arking, 1991, p. 249 and Chapters 6, 10, 12, 13.
46. Shakespeare, *Hamlet*, V.v.17.
47. Hayflick and Moorehead, 1961. For reviews, see also Hayflick, 1965, and Goldstein, 1990.
48. Brown, Zebrower, and Kieras, 1990.
49. Martin, 1993.
50. Ibid.
51. Arking, 1991, p. 369; addition of the word "molecules" with his permission, 1993.
52. Lamb, 1977.
53. See Rose, 1991; particularly Chapter 5, for a cogent and thoughtful explanation of the problems of understanding aging from an evolutionary viewpoint.
54. Comfort, 1979, p. 16; quoted in Arking, 1991, p. 3.

Chapter 3: The Clock

1. With some exceptions. For example, mature red cells have no chromosomes, some cerebellar neurons have twice the normal number, and some cells have several nuclei.
2. Sen and Gilbert, 1992; Laughlan et al., 1994.
3. Moyzis, 1991.
4. Blackburn, 1990.
5. Biessmann and Mason, 1992.
6. Other simple DNA sequences can also exist interspersed with this degenerate telomerelike DNA. See Allshire, 1989; Counter et al., 1992; Levy et al., 1992.
7. Or ribonucleoprotein molecules. See the review and discussion by Weiner, 1988, for his rationale for suggesting that telomerase is an ancient (pre-DNA) enzyme.
8. Weiner, 1988; Orgel, 1994.
9. Although reverse transcriptase comes immediately to mind, given the current epidemic of deaths from and interest in understanding and curing AIDS.
10. Muller, 1938. Cited in Biessmann and Mason, 1992.
11. See the account in Watson, 1968.
12. Greider, 1991; McClintock, 1941.
13. Watson, 1972.
14. Olovnikov, 1971.
15. Olovnikov, 1973.
16. For example, Blackburn and Chiou, 1981.
17. Cooke and Smith, 1986.
18. Hastie et al., 1990.
19. This discussion largely follows and is indebted to Biessmann and Mason, 1992, who may disagree with the uses to which I have put their superb review. See also Chikashige et al. 1994; Blackburn and Szostak, 1984; and Zakian, 1989.
20. Greider and Blackburn, 1985.
21. Telomerases—the enzymes that add TTAGGGs to the telomeres in your germ cells—differ for each base sequence (for example your own TTAGGG), but they can add sequences, in vitro, onto the telomeres from almost any organism, no matter what their normal sequence is supposed to be. When telomerase is used on the "wrong" telomere (from the "wrong" organism), it adds the

20. Lindsey et al., 1991.

21. Conley, 1974.

22. Potten and Morris, 1988; Hastie et al., 1990.

23. Hastie et al., 1990. See also Vaziri et al., 1994.

24. Actually, mature red blood cells don't have normal telomeres or even nuclei for that matter. Both stem cells in the marrow and immature red blood cells do, however, and most of this discussion assumes we are discussing these rather than mature red cells.

25. Vaziri et al., 1993.

26. Coffin, 1995; Ho et al., 1995; Wei et al., 1995.

27. Counter et al., 1995.

28. Bender et al., 1989.

29. Chang and Harley, 1995.

30. Counter et al., 1992.

31. Hastie et al., 1990.

32. Morin, 1989.

33. Counter et al., 1992

34. Ross, 1986, cited in Chang and Harley, 1995.

35. E.g., Moore, 1981; discussed in Chang and Harley, 1995.

36. Discussed in Chang and Harley, 1995.

37. Cooper, Cooke, and Dzau, 1994.

38. Robbins, 1974, Chapter 15.

39. Chang and Harley, 1995.

40. Moss and Benditt, 1973.

41. Chang and Harley, 1995.

42. Danny, the oldest living progeric as I write this, is twenty-one. I was privileged to meet him and his mother in Florida in June of 1995.

43. Goldstein, 1978; pp. 171–224; Mills and Weiss, 1990.

44. Allsopp et al., 1992.

45. Discussed in Allsopp et al., 1992; see also Mills and Weiss, 1990.

46. At least by mid-1995.

47. Martin, 1993.

48. C-fos, for example, a common cell enzyme, doesn't fall to the same degree; Martin, 1993.

49. Vaziri et al., 1993.

50. Coffin, 1995; Ho et al., 1995; Wei et al., 1995.

51. See PCT Patent Publication No. 95/13382. An alternative explana-

tion of the final failure of the immune system in AIDS, the "Diversity Threshold Model" of Nowak and McMichael, 1995, is not at all inconsistent with the comments offered here, but both of these theories may be necessary to explain the clinical outcome.

52. Heinlein, 1958.
53. Especially since there was no "weeding out" of descendants with short life spans.
54. C. B. Harley and B. Villeponteau, personal communication, 1993.
55. Goldstein, 1990.

Chapter 5: Time Runs Out

1. The best single discussion of this is probably in Cooper, Cooke, and Dzau, 1994.
2. Cooper, Cooke, and Dzau, 1994.
3. For example, they no longer produce as much prostacyclin or endothelial-derived growth factor (nitric oxide), both of which inhibit many of the changes that occur in the vascular disease of aging. For a detailed discussion of these and other changes that occur with aging of endothelial cells—and which play a major role in vessel disease—see Cooper, Cooke, and Dzau, 1994.
4. Lakatta, 1994, p. 500
5. Ibid, p. 505; see also Hayflick, 1994, e.g., p. 144.
6. A good quick overview of glial function—and reference to the problem of excitatory transmitters and the damage to neurons—is provided by Travis, 1995.
7. Including glial-cell-line derived neurotrophic factor (GDNF), nerve growth factor (NGF), CEP-1347 (along with other members of the same family of compounds), and an unknown but growing number of other trophic factors.
8. See both Fackelmann's, 1995, and Barinaga's, 1995, reviews for quick overviews of some of the recent work.
9. Samorajski, 1976.
10. Sturrock, 1976; Vernadakis, 1975. The conclusion that they shorten their telomeres has not, as I write this, been confirmed. We do know that the telomeres of cortical neurons do not shorten (Allsopp et al., in press). The glia/neuron ratio is 10/1 overall and lower in the cortical tissue on which Allsopp et al.'s work is based.

To the extent that their telomere measurements reflect glial cells in addition to neurons, there is no evidence that these cortical glial cells divide at all.

11. Almost none of your neurons divide after birth. See, for example, Rakic, 1985.

12. Tholey and Ledig, 1990; Streit and Kincaid-Colton, 1995.

13. Particularly inflammation in microglia. See, for example, Pennisi, 1993.

14. The literature on supportive trophic factors, necessary to the survival and function of neurons, is growing rapidly. For a quick sketch of some recent developments, see Nishi, 1994.

15. Hendrix, 1974.

16. Arking, 1991, p. 162.

17. Baime, Nelson, and Castell, 1994. There is some evidence that crypt cells in the gastrointestinal tract may express small amounts of telomerase (J. Shay, personal communication, 1995). Their telomeres may still shorten with each division, albeit more slowly than other cells.

18. No one really knows yet. Information bearing on this argument can be found in Beck's (1994, p. 616) discussion of work on aging renal blood flow.

19. This discussion doesn't even touch on loss of trabecula, which may not be replaceable (Baylink and Jennings, 1994, p. 883). On the other hand, osteoblasts built them once and might be capable of doing so again. This is not necessarily parallel to the problem of structure damage and loss of structural information (such as in the lung, where rebuilding of the structure may not occur): Trabeculae are remodeled throughout life as it is.

20. Arking, 1991, p. 208.

21. Gregerman and Katz, 1994, p. 809.

22. The distinction is clear biochemically, slightly less clear functionally, and only roughly true anatomically.

23. The best discussion of this topic occupied an entire issue of *Experimental Gerontology* (1994; Vol. 29, No. 3/4). See particularly Gosden and Faddy, 1994; Wise et al., 1994; Judd and Fourney, 1994.

24. And is undergoing a revival. See, for example, *Time* magazine, January 23, 1995, p. 52. Also Seachrist, "Hormone Mimics Fabled Fountain of Youth," 1995.

25. There are a number of articles suggesting that it helps protect against mammary tumors, particularly in rats, but it may have other benefits as well. See Seachrist, op. cit.
26. Sapolsky, 1992.
27. Terry and Halter, 1994.
28. Pierpaoli, Regelson, and Fabris, 1994; Pierpaoli, Regelson, and Colman, 1995.
29. Although melatonin might still extend the *average* life span, judging from the animal studies. Remember, however, that historically similar claims have been made for DHEA and growth hormone, as well as—to a less radical extent—thyroid hormone, testosterone, and estrogen. All of these claims are accurate to a degree: Each compound reverses certain of the outcomes of aging, but with differing, and uncertain, risks.
30. DiGiovanna, 1994, Chapter 15.

Chapter 6: Turning Back the Clock
1. See, for example, Walters, 1991; Wivel and Walters, 1993.
2. Wivel and Walters, 1993, p. 533.
3. See the relevant patent application (PCT Publication No. 93/23572) regarding telomere extension and "capping."
4. At least the RNA component of telomerase is apparently a single-copy gene localized on the distal quarter of the long arm of chromosome three; Feng et al., 1995.
5. Feng et al., 1995.
6. Liposomes are small "balls" with walls made of lipids, which could contain genetic, or other material, for delivery to cells. For a recent overview, see Lasic and Papahadjopoulos, 1995. Dendrimers are another possible delivery system; see Service, 1995.
7. For a bit of appropriate optimism and more information about retroviral vectors (which is what we are actually discussing here), see Bushman, 1995; Marshall, 1995; Anderson, 1995.
8. The telomerase gene is repressed as part of the distinction between germ and somatic cells, probably at the outset of the developmental path from fertilized germ cell to differentiated somatic cell. Differentiation itself, as it causes the expression of some genes and the emphatic suppression of others, is probably indissolvably linked to telomerase suppression: Expressing telomerase might jeopardize

the pattern of gene expression appropriate to each differentiated, somatic cell.

9. This bald statement turns on the definition of "malignant." See Kim et al., 1994, and Hiyama et al., 1995, for examples of cancer cells that express little or no telomerase.

10. Personal communication, 1995.

11. Feng et al., 1995.

12. And probably immune function, energy levels, etc.

13. See, for example, Gillman et al., 1995, and Voelker, 1995.

14. See both Herbert 1994, and references for a place to start and an interesting perspective on this issue. A concise and balanced perspective is provided by Dr. Bruce Ames (famous for his careful assessment of relative risks of carcinogenesis) in which he discusses what we know (and what we don't) about vitamins, antioxidants, and their relationship to heart disease (Voelker, 1995).

15. Herbert, 1994. See particularly notes 2, 3, 5, and 6.

16. Actually, a single copy of the gene for the RNA component of telomerase is found on the distal quarter of the long arm of chromosome three; Feng et al., 1995.

17. This is an estimate with several caveats. It includes the cost of the drug itself, but not the delivery costs (nurse or physician charges, office overhead, or hospitalization charges if applicable). It is based on U.S. 1995 dollars, and assumes that there are no major side effects and unexpected liability costs. The estimate is based on similar development and patient costs of current drugs such as azithromycin, TPA, Epogen (erythropoietin), etc. Finally, the initial cost of telomerase induction will be higher, perhaps $10,000 U.S. 1995 dollars, until, as safety and efficacy are confirmed, more patients opt for the therapy and the final costs stabilize within the range quoted here.

18. This figure is the estimated number of newly diagnosed cancer cases in the United States in 1994. It includes approximately 800,000 skin cancers and 1.2 million other sites. *World Almanac,* 1995.

19. This figure is elusive for several reasons. The entire population might serve as the first approximation, since everyone ages. From this, we have to subtract those who die young of whatever cause (only half the population in most developed countries achieves the

average life span, usually about seventy-five, but many will want to be treated well before the age of forty) and those who would decline therapy. The final figure will be large, but is hard to predict accurately.

20. Courtesy of Greg Baird, Corporate Communication, Genentech, 1995.

21. Ibid.

22. Except within the legal confines of patent law.

23. Kessler and Feiden, 1995.

24. The current best guess is that the IND (Investigational New Drug) criteria will be met before 2000 and that the NDA (New Drug Application) will be approved by 2005. Compare this with the 6.5 year average for standard NDAs, or 2.5–4.5 years under the FDA's "accelerated procedures" (Kessler and Feiden, 1995).

Chapter 7: The Rewound Clock

1. Muscle cells themselves don't divide, but they do have "satellite cells" from which new muscle cells can form. The practical significance in reversing aging is anyone's guess, but it does provide grounds for optimism for those inclined toward it.

2. Herbert et al., 1995.

3. Adler and Nagel, 1994.

4. For example, Hiyama et al., 1995.

5. Animal trials of telomerase inhibitors (for example, antisense RNA to telomerase; Feng et al., 1995) will begin at Memorial Sloan Kettering Cancer Institute with the aid of a $2 million grant from the National Cancer Institute in September 1995.

6. Feng et al., 1995.

7. At the Memorial Sloan Kettering Cancer Institute.

8. See Harley et al., 1994, for an interesting short discussion of this.

9. The length of the telomere in cancer cells varies a good deal. Although shorter than in normal cells, it is not reliably so. See the discussion in Hiyama et al., 1995.

10. Even in the case of germ cells, any effect should be on sperm cells only, as ova have already finished dividing prenatally.

11. Compare this discussion with Harley et al., 1994.

12. Counter et al., 1995.

13. For example, terminal restriction fragments were measured in Has-

tie et al., 1990; see also Harley et al., 1994. Haber, 1995, is cautiously optimistic in his editorial on this work.

14. See both Kim et al., 1994, and Hiyama et al., 1995.

15. Harley et al., 1994.

16. Blackburn, 1990.

17. Malaria, schistosomiasis, filariasis, African trypanosomiasis, Chagas's disease, and leishmaniasis. Gallagher, Marx, and Hines, 1994.

18. This information is both from her talk "Development of Neurotrophic Approaches to Alzheimer's Disease" (given June 8, 1995, in Danvers, Massachusetts, at the Cambridge Healthtech Institute's conference "Alzheimer's Disease: The Promise of New Therapeutics") and from private communication, 1995.

19. See Finch, 1994; Mann, 1993.

20. See Corder et al., 1995, for a quick introduction to this concept and two self-explanatory figures.

21. Alzheimer's disease is strongly linked to chromosome 21 (site of the amyloid precursor gene), but there is also a clear linkage to both chromosomes 14 and 19 (the latter being the site of the gene for apolipoprotein E).

22. For example, beta amyloid and tau proteins.

23. Arking, 1991, pp. 195, 197ff., 361.

24. Baylink and Jennings, 1994, p. 889.

25. Or similar hormonal therapies.

26. The etiology of adult onset diabetes remains a source of contention. See Weir, 1995; Pimenta et al., 1995.

27. Goldberg and Coon, 1994, p. 824.

28. See Arking, 1991, p. 71, for a discussion of lens changes.

29. Privileged communication, 1994.

30. Which is technically a chromosomal rather than a genetic disease in any case.

31. Enzyme defects as well as many others whose etiology we are ignorant of are obvious candidates for the list: sickle-cell disease, Tay-Sachs disease, Turner's syndrome, Von Willebrand disease, and by now hundreds of others.

32. Harman, 1993, p. 209.

33. Oogonia, actually. See the short discussion regarding telomerase and the female germ line in Harley et al., 1994.

34. Counter et al., 1995.

35. On the other hand, if these cells *do* use a telomeric clock to determine when to close the epiphyseal plates, then we'll have to be careful not to use telomere therapy on patients whose growth plates are still active.

36. The figures assume 1959 United States actuarial data, averaged for sex, and they depend heavily on the age because age determines accidental death rate so strongly. As you might guess, accidental death rates peak in the teens and early twenties (when we are prone to take chances?), nadir out in the thirties, and then slowly rise again as reaction times and healing abilities fall off (and telomeres shorten). The accidental death rate for 99-year-olds, for example, is 15/1000, but for 69-year-olds is only 1/1000, and for 39-year-olds is only .39/1000. These figures are equivalent to death rates of 0.985000, 0.99900, and 0.99961 per year, respectively. Using the formula:

(death rate) ^{X} = .5

where .5 represents median (50th percentile) survival and x represents the median age at death, then if we remove all sources of nonaccidental death, the human life span still depends critically on which death rate we choose. The median life spans (based on 1959 death statistics, averaged for lifestyle, genetic influences, sex, etc.) would be:

> using the 39-year-olds' death rate——1777 years
> using the 69-year-olds' death rate——693 years
> using the 99-year-olds' death rate—— 46 years

Presumably, lengthening the telomeres would have the effect of moving your death rate closer to a 39-year-old's than an older—and higher—death rate based only on chronological age. Age-specific death rate information from McAlpine, 1995.

37. It might not be independent at all. Perhaps as the cells age from telomere changes, they become less able to oxidize the lipids that then form lipofuscin. Arking (1991, p. 349) points out that these pigments arise when "antioxidant defense systems begin to decline." It is possible that telomere therapy might prevent, or even reverse, the problem. The only way to be sure is to wait and see.

38. These figures grow from the literature and from discussions with Dr. Michael West; personal communication, 1995. An entire con-

ference explored these issues in San Antonio in October 1995 but figures are still hard to come by.

39. Evidence suggests they originally evolved as independent organisms that later became accustomed to living inside other cells. Now they are dependent on us and we are very dependent on them.

40. What if we could make copies of this information, however? Suppose we might "back up" our brains, much as we interminably back up our computer files. This notion has been repeatedly explored in science fiction already. Perhaps I am too pessimistic.

Chapter 8: Telling Times

1. Those working on this therapy aim to have the New Drug Application approved for use of a telomerase inhibitor within ten years. Private communication, 1995.

2. Hayflick, 1994, p. 336.

3. Roush, 1994; Keyfitz, 1993.

4. See especially Livi-Bacci, 1989; but also Piel, 1994; Roush, 1994.

5. Livi-Bacci, 1989, p. 104. There is considerable disagreement on these figures. Compare the transition time given for Sweden according to Livi-Bacci (150 years) with that given by Roush, 1994 (a negative number).

6. This discussion ignores the issue of population momentum, which is more appropriately addressed in any text on population, such as Livi-Bacci, 1989.

7. Livi-Bacci, 1989, p. 122.

8. For a quick perspective on the argument that sufficient economic improvement creates environmental improvement, see Arrow et al., 1995.

9. Kirkland, 1994.

10. If we assume that everyone between ages eighteen and sixty-four works, then 66.7 percent of the population works. If we assume that everyone sixty-five years or older is retired, then 12.6 percent of the population is retired. This gives us a first approximation of five workers per retired person in the United States (Banks, 1995).

11. If we assume that everyone between ages eighteen and sixty-four will work, then 56.7 percent of the population will be working. If we assume that everyone sixty-five years or older retires, then 20.2 percent of the population will have retired. This gives us a first

approximation of fewer than three workers per retired person in the United States (Banks, 1995).

12. And how well the investment does.

13. Dychtwald and Flower, 1990, p. 32.

14. It happened in the case of the current CEO of McDonald's Corporation, Michael Quinlan. Almost the same case occurred when Edward Rens, the current president of McDonald's International, started as a "new member."

15. This will be true unless the demand for services increases. As the use of current medical services falls with the advent of telomere therapy, rather than paying a smaller premium, subscribers might demand more services (not affected by telomere therapy) such as psychiatric or genetic treatments. In addition, the advent of telomere therapy might increase social stress and thus the frequency of trauma (murder, suicide, etc.). Medicare costs will diminish only to the extent that we assume the current pattern of use will continue. The author is indebted to Banks, 1995, for clarifying this point.

16. In all of these examples, training is measured from acquisition of a high school diploma to the time at which the trainee has paid for the costs of training. Physicians, for example, typically take almost ten years after residency to pay off their loans. The issue of arbitrary certification (M.D., for example) is not explicit in this discussion—and this is not the forum for such a discussion—but is implicit in the cost of training many workers and substantially increases those costs. Milton Friedman and other economists have written on this issue in some detail. Acknowledgment to Banks, 1995.

17. This example is real; the result of a venture capitalist's evaluation of a company prior to purchase. Private communication, 1994.

18. But this proportion is likely to decrease in the future in any case, regardless of telomere therapy, as technological advances—robotics, for example—account for more of the cost of production and labor accounts for less. In short, the capital-to-labor ratio will go up. Acknowledgment to Banks, 1995.

19. As Dwayne Banks, a professor of economics at Berkeley, would have me put it: "As productivity increases, per unit labor costs decline, workers' real wages will increase, *ceteris paribus*." (Banks, 1995).

20. Actually, while it is a real gain, inefficient and unnecessary sectors of the economy *will* suffer. The health insurance industry and portions of our current medical system will shrink and many workers with extensive—and expensive—training will be unemployed.

21. This assumes that a great many things do not change, for example how people spend their money and where they do so. If everyone moves to Palo Alto, the price of real estate will climb and with it the cost of living there. The conclusion that reduced labor costs will reduce the cost of living is true on the average and only to the extent that other market and economic factors don't change, which they are likely to do in unpredictable ways even without telomere therapy. Acknowledgment to Banks, 1995.

22. The author thanks Dwayne Banks (1995) for his comments regarding the issue raised in this paragraph.

23. Actually real estate is peculiar. Real estate isn't so much a fixed resource (the amount of land on earth) as it is a matter of relative worth. Certain tracts of land are suited to agriculture or home building and others are not. As the costs of real estate rise, a certain amount of previously unusable land becomes worthwhile until the point that mosquito-infested swampland or forty-five-degree-angle mountain slopes are used for farming or building. The fact remains, however, that prices go up *throughout* the spectrum of properties from prime real estate to swampland and rocky slopes. Arguments about real estate beyond the earth are fascinating, but have no effect on the conclusion: Real estate acts like a fixed resource.

24. From his lecture at Johns Hopkins University, February 22, 1904, quoted in Cushing, 1925.

25. New York Stock Exchange figures show that 51 percent of all American households in 1995 held individual stock shares (NYSE, private communication, 1995); approximately 90 percent of households in 1995 with total gross income over $30,000 per year owned shares in a mutual fund (courtesy of the Research Department, Oppenheimer Mutual, 1995)—and neither of these figures includes all households in which someone owns stock through a pension plan rather than personally.

26. Smith, 1993.

27. "Matrix" families in Dychtwald and Flower's term, 1990.

28. *World Almanac*, 1992.
29. Amnesty International, 1994.
30. Quoted in Horgan, 1994, p. 33.
31. *World Almanac*, 1992, p. 725.
32. Private conversation between Michael West and Francis Schaeffer; reported to me by Michael West, 1993.
33. Jakobovits, 1989.
34. Bleich, 1989.
35. Ibid. 1989.
36. Courtesy of Professor Aziz Sachedina, 1994.
37. For a useful and short discussion, see Desai, 1988.
38. Desai, 1988.
39. Morgan, 1995.
40. In a private discussion with Roshi Philip Kapleau in 1973, he told me that it didn't matter whether or not one accepted Buddhism within one's lifetime, "because there will always be other lifetimes."
41. Desai, 1988.

BIBLIOGRAPHY

Adler, W.H., and J.E. Nagel. "Clinical Immunology and Aging." Chapter 5 in Hazzard, W.R., et al. *Principles of Geriatric Medicine and Gerontology*, 3rd ed. New York: McGraw-Hill, 1994.

Allshire, R.C., M. Dempster, and N.D. Hastie. "Human Telomeres Contain at Least Three Types of G-Rich Repeat Distributed Nonrandomly." *Nucleic Acids Research*, Vol. 17 (1989), p. 4611.

Allsopp, R.C., and C.B. Harley. "Evidence for a Critical Telomere Length in Senescent Human Fibroblasts." *Experimental-Cell Research*, Vol. 219 (1995), pp. 130–136.

———, et al. "Telomere Shortening Is Associated with Cell Division *In Vitro* and *In Vivo*." *Experimental Cell Research*, Vol. 220 (1995), pp. 194–200.

———, et al. "Telomere Length Predicts Replicative Capacity of Human Fibroblasts." *Proceedings of the National Academy of Science*, Vol. 89, No. 21 (1992), pp. 10, 114–18.

Amenta, F. *Aging of the Autonomic Nervous System*. Boca Raton, Fla.: CRC Press, 1993.

Amnesty International. *The Death Penalty List of Abolitionist and Retentionist Countries (December 1, 1993)*. External distribution. London: International Secretariat, 1994.

Anderson, W.F. "Gene Therapy." *Scientific American*, September 1995, pp. 124–128.

Arking, R. *Biology of Aging—Observations and Principles*. Englewood Cliffs, N.J.: Prentice-Hall, 1991.

Arrow, K., et al. "Economic Growth, Carrying Capacity, and the Environment." *Science*, Vol. 268 (1995), pp. 520–21.

Baime M.J., J.B. Nelson, and D.O. Castell. "Aging of the Gastrointestinal system." Chapter 58 in Hazzard et al., op. cit.

Banks, D. (assistant professor of economics at the University of California at Berkeley). Personal communication, 1995.

Barinaga, M. "Researchers Broaden the Attack on Parkinson's Disease." *Science*, Vol. 267 (1995), pp. 455–56.

Baylink, D.J., and J.C. Jennings. "Calcium and Bone Homeostasis and Changes with Aging." Chapter 75 in Hazzard et al., op. cit.

Beck, L.H. "Aging Changes in Renal Function." Chapter 54 in Hazzard et al., op. cit.

Beck W.S. "Human Body." In *The Encylopedia Americana*. Danbury, Conn.: Grolier, 1983.

Bender, M.A., et al. "Chromosomal Aberration and Sister-Chromatid Exchange Frequencies in Peripheral Blood Lymphocytes of a Large Human Population Sample." *Mutation Research*, Vol. 212 (1989), pp. 149–54.

Berg, J.M., H. Karlinsky, and A.J. Holland. *Alzheimer Disease, Down Syndrome, and Their Relationship*. New York: Oxford University Press, 1994.

Biessmann, H., and J.M. Mason. "Genetics and Molecular Biology of Telomeres." *Advances in Genetics*, Vol. 30 (1992), pp. 185–249.

———, S.B. Carter, and J.M. Mason. "Chromosome Ends in Drosophila Without Telomeric DNA Sequences." *Proceedings of the National Academy of Science*, Vol. 87 (1990), pp. 1758–61.

Blackburn E.H. "Telomeres: Structure and Synthesis." *Journal of Biological Chemistry*, Vol. 265, No. 11 (1990), pp. 5919–21.

———, and S.S. Chiou. "Non-nucleosomal Packaging of a Tandemly Repeated DNA Sequence at Termini of Extrachromosomal DNA Coding for rRNA in Tetrahymena." *Proceedings of the National Academy of Science*, Vol. 78, No. 4 (April 1981), pp. 2263–67.

———, and J.W. Szostak. "The Molecular Structure of Centromeres and Telomeres." *Annual Review of Biochemistry*, Vol. 53 (1984), pp. 163–94.

Bleich, J.D. "Artificial Insemination and Genetic Engineering." Chapter 7 in Steinberg, op. cit.

Brown, W.T., M. Zebrower, and F.J. Kieras. "Progeria: A Genetic D Disease Model of Premature Aging." Chapter 29 in *Genetic Effects on Aging II*, ed. D.E. Harrison. Caldwell, N.J.: Telford Press, 1990.

Bushman, F. "Targeting Retroviral Integration." *Science*, Vol. 267 (1995), pp. 1443–44.

Chang, E. and C.B. Harley. "Telomere Length as a Measure of Replicative Histories in Human Vascular Tissues." *Proceedings of the National Academy of Science*, Vol. 92 (1995).

Chikashige, Y., et al. "Telomere-Led Premeiotic Chromosome Movement in Fission Yeast." *Science*, Vol. 264 (1994), pp. 270–73.

Coffin, J.M. "HIV Population Dynamics in Vivo: Implications for Genetic Variation, Pathogenesis, and Therapy." *Science*, Vol. 267 (1995), pp. 483–89.

Cohen J. "Getting All Turned Around over the Origins of Life on Earth." *Science*, Vol. 267 (1995), pp. 1265–66.

Comfort, A. *Ageing: The Biology of Senescence*, 2nd ed. New York: Holt, Rinehart and Winston, 1964.

———. *Ageing: The Biology of Senescence*, 3rd ed. New York: Holt, Rinehart and Winston, 1979.

Conley, C.L. "The Blood." Chapter 44 in Mountcastle, V.B. *Medical Physiology*, 13th ed. St. Louis: C.V. Mosby, 1974.

Cooke, H.J., and B.A. Smith. "Variability at the Telomeres of Human X/Y

Pseudoautosomal Region." *Cold Spring Harbor Symposia on Quantitative Biology.* Vol. 51 (1986), pp. 213–19.

Cooper, L.T., J.P. Cooke, and V.J. Dzau. "The Vasculopathy of Aging." *Journal of Gerontology, Biological Sciences,* Vol. 49 (1994), pp. B191–96.

Corder, E.H., et al. "Letters: The Apolipoprotein E *E4* Allele and Sex-Specific Risk of Alzheimer's Disease." *Journal of the American Medical Association,* Vol. 273 (1995), pp. 373–74.

Counter, C.M., et al. "Telomere Shortening Associated with Chromosome Instability Is Arrested in Immortal Cells Which Express Telomerase Activity." *European Molecular Biology Organization Journal,* Vol. II (1992), pp. 1921–29.

————, et al. "Telomerase Activity in Human Ovarian Carcinoma." *Proceedings of the National Academy of Science,* Vol. 91 (1994), pp. 2900–4.

————, et al. "Telomerase Activity in Normal Leukocytes and in Hematologic Malignancies." *Blood,* Vol. 85 (1995), pp. 2315–20.

Cross, S.H., et al. "Cloning of Human Telomeres by Complementation in Yeast." *Nature,* Vol. 338 (1989), pp. 771–74.

Cushing, H. *The Life of Sir William Osler.* Oxford, U.K.: Clarendon Press, 1925.

Cutler, R.G. "Antioxidants and Longevity of Mammalian Species." In *Molecular Biology of Aging,* ed. A.D. Woodhead, A.D. Blackett, and A. Hollaender. New York: Plenum Press, 1985.

de Lange, T., et al. "Structure and Viability of Human Chromosome Ends." *Molecular Cellular Biology,* Vol. 10 (1990), pp. 518–27.

Desai, P.N. "Medical Ethics in India." *Journal of Medicine and Philosophy,* Vol. 23 (1988), pp. 231–55.

DiGiovanna, A.G. *Human Aging: Biological Perspectives.* New York: McGraw-Hill, 1994.

D'Mello, N.P., and S.M. Jazwinski. "Telomere Length Constancy During Aging of Saccharomyces Cerevisiae." *Journal of Bacteriology,* Vol. 173 (1991), pp. 6709–13.

Dychtwald, K., and J. Flower. *Age Wave.* New York: Bantam, 1990.

Fackelmann, K. "Protein Protects, Restores Neurons." *Science News,* Vol. 147 (1995), p. 52.

Feeney, G. "Fertility Decline in East Asia." *Science,* Vol. 266 (1994), pp. 1518–23.

Fefer, A. "Diseases of the Spleen and Reticuloendothelial System." Chapter 320 in *Harrison's Principles of Internal Medicine,* 8th ed. New York: McGraw-Hill, 1977.

Feng, J., et al. "The RNA Component of Human Telomerase." *Science,* Vol. 269 (1995), pp 1236–1241.

Finch, C.E. *Longevity, Senescence, and the Genome.* Chicago: University of Chicago Press, 1990.

————. "The Evolution of Ovarian Oocyte Decline with Aging and Possible

Relationships to Down Syndrome and Alzheimer Disease." *Experimental Gerontology*, Vol. 29 (1994), pp. 299–304.

Floyd, R.A. "Basic Free Radical Biochemistry." Chapter 3 in Yu, B.P. *Free Radicals in Aging*. Boca Raton, Fla.: CRC Press, 1993.

Fraga, C.G., et al. "Oxidative Damage to DNA During Aging: 8-Hydroxy-2'-Deoxyguanosine in Rat Organ DNA and Urine." *Proceedings of the National Academy of Science*, Vol. 87 (1990), p. 4533.

Galeano, E. *Open Veins of Latin America—Five Centuries of the Pillage of a Continent*. New York: Monthly Review Press, 1973.

Gallagher, R.B., J. Marx and P.J. Hines. *Science*, Vol. 264 (1994), p. 1827.

Gillman, M.W., et al. "Protective Effect of Fruits and Vegetables on Development of Stroke in Men." *Journal of the American Medical Association*, Vol. 273 (1995), pp. 1113–17.

Goldberg, A.J., and P.J. Coon. "Diabetes Mellitus and Glucose Metabolism in the Elderly." Chapter 71 in Hazzard et al., op. cit.

———, et al. "Protein Synthetic Fidelity in Aging Human Fibroblasts." *Advances in Experimental-Medicine and Biology*, Vol. 190 (1985), pp. 495–508.

Goldstein, S., In *Genetics of Aging*, ed. E.L. Schneider. New York: Plenum, 1978.

———. "Replicative Senescence: The Human Fibroblast Comes of Age." *Science*, Vol. 249 (1990), pp. 1129–33.

Gosden R.G., and M.J. Faddy. "Ovarian Aging, Follicular Depletion, and Steroidogenesis." *Experimental Gerontology*, Vol. 29 (1991), pp. 265–74.

Gottschling, D.E., et al. "Position Effect at S. Cerevisiae Telomeres: Reversible Repression of Pol II Transcription." *Cell*, Vol. 63 (1990), pp. 751–62.

Gregerman, R.I., and M.S. Katz. "Thyroid Diseases." Chapter 70 in Hazzard et al; op. cit.

———, and E.H. Blackburn. "Identification of a Specific Telomere Terminal Transferase Activity in Tetrahymena Extracts." *Cell*, Vol. 43, No. 2 (December 1985) pp. 405–13.

Greider, C.W. "Telomerase Is Processive." *Mol. Cell. Biol.*, Vol. 11, No. 9 (1991), pp. 4572–80.

Griffiths, T.D. "DNA Synthesis, Cell Progression and Aging in Human Diploid Fibroblasts." In Roy, A.K, and B. Chatterjee. *Molecular Basis of Aging*. New York: Academic Press, 1984, pp. 95–118.

Haber, D.A. "Telomeres, Cancer, and Immortality." *New England Journal of Medicine*, Vol. 332 (1995), pp. 95–96.

Harley, C.B. "Biology and Evolution of Aging: Implications for Basic Gerontological Health Research." *Canadian Journal of Aging*, Vol. 7 (1988), pp. 100–13.

———. "Telomere Loss: Mitotic Clock or Genetic Time Bomb?" *Mutation Research*, Vol. 256 (1991), pp. 271–82.

———, A.B. Futcher, and C.W. Greider. "Telomeres Shorten During Aging of Human Fibroblasts." *Nature*, Vol. 345, No. 6274 (1990), pp. 458–60.

———, et al. "Loss of Repetitious DNA in Proliferating Somatic Cells May

Be Due to Unequal Recombination." *Journal of Theoretical Biology*, Vol. 94, No. 1 (1982), pp. 1–12.

——, et al. "Telomerase, Cell Immortality, and Cancer." *Cold Spring Harbor Symposia on Quantitative Biology*, Vol. 59 (1994), pp. 307–15.

Harman, D. "Free Radicals and Age-Related Diseases." Chapter 9 in Yu, op. cit.

Hastie, N.D., et al. "Telomere Reduction in Human Colorectal Carcinoma and with Ageing." *Nature*, Vol. 346 (1990), pp. 866–68.

Hayflick, L. "The Limited *In Vitro* Lifetime of Human Diploid Cell Strains." *Experimental Cell Research*, Vol. 37 (1965), pp. 614–36.

——. *How and Why We Age*. New York: Ballantine Books, 1994.

——, and P.S. Moorehead. "The Limited *In Vitro* Lifetime of Human Diploid Cell Strains." *Experimental Aging Research*, Vol. 25 (1961), pp. 585–621.

Hazzard, W.R., et al. *Principles of Geriatric Medicine and Gerontology*, 3rd ed. New York: McGraw-Hill, 1994.

Hebert, L.E., et al. "Age-Specific Incidence of Alzheimer's Disease in a Community Population." *Journal of the American Medical Association*, Vol. 273 (1995), pp. 1354–59.

Heinlein, R.A. *Methuselah's Children*. New York: Signet, 1958.

Hendrix, T.R. "The Absorptive Function of the Alimentary Canal." Chapter 50 in Mountcastle, op. cit.

Herbert, V. "Antioxidants, Pro-oxidants, and Their Effects." *Journal of the American Medical Association*, Vol. 272 (1994), p. 1659.

Hiyama, E., et al. "Correlating Telomerase Activity Levels with Human Neuroblastoma Outcomes." *Nature Medicine*, Vol. 1 (1995), pp. 249–54.

Ho, D.D., et al. "Rapid Turnover of Plasma Virions and CD-4 Lymphocytes on HIV-1 Injection," Vol. 373 (1995), p. 123.

Horgan, J. "Profile: The Final Limit, Subrahmanyan Chandrasekhar." *Scientific American*, March 1994, p. 33.

Jakobovits, L.I. In Steinberg, A. "The European Colloquium on Medical Ethics," op. cit.

Jitsukawa, M., and C. Djerassi. "Birth Control in Japan: Realities and Prognosis." *Science*, Vol. 265 (1994), pp. 1048–51.

Johnson, J.E., et al. *Free Radicals, Aging and Degenerative Diseases*. New York: Liss, 1986.

Judd, H.L., and N. Fournet. "Changes of Ovarian Hormonal Function with Aging." *Experimental Gerontology*, Vol. 29 (1994), pp. 285–98.

Katz, M.K., and W.G. Robison, Jr. "Nutritional Influences on Autoxidation, Lipofuscin Accumulation, and Aging." In Johnson et al., op. cit.

Kessler, D., and K.L. Feiden. "Faster Evaluation of Vital Drugs." *Scientific American*, March 1995, pp. 48–54.

Keyfitz, N. "Population." *Grolier's Electronic Encyclopedia*, 1993.

Kim, N.W., et al. "Specific Association of Human Telomerase Activity with Immortal Cells and Cancer." *Science*, Vol. 266 (1994), pp. 2011–14.

——, et al. "Letters" (response). *Science*, Vol. 268 (1995), pp. 1116–17.

Kipling, D. *The Telomere*. New York: Oxford University Press, 1995.

——, and H.J. Cooke. "Hypervariable Ultra-Long Telomeres in Mice." *Nature*, Vol. 397 (1990), pp. 400–402.

Kirkland, R.I. "Why We Will Live Longer . . . and What It Will Mean." *Fortune*, February 1994.

Kreil, G. "Conversion of L- to D-Amino Acids: A Posttranslational Reaction." *Science*, Vol. 266 (1994), pp. 996–97.

Lakatta, E.G. "Alterations in Circulatory Function." Chapter 43 in Hazzard et al., op. cit.

Lamb, M.J. *Biology of Ageing*. New York: Wiley Halsted Press, 1977.

Lasic, D.D., and D. Papahadjopoulos. "Liposomes Revisited." *Science*, Vol. 267 (1995), pp. 1275–76.

Laughlan, G., et al. "The High-Resolution Crystal Structure of a Parallel-Stranded Guanine Tetraplex." *Science*, Vol. 265 (1994), pp. 520–24.

Levy, M.Z., et al. "Telomere End-Replication Problem and Cell Aging." *Journal of Molecular Biology*, Vol. 225 (1992), pp. 951–60.

Lindsey J., et al. "In Vivo Loss of Telomeric Repeats with Age in Humans." *Mutation Research*, Vol. 256 (1991), pp. 45–48.

Livi-Bacci, M. *A Concise History of World Population*. Cambridge, Mass.: Blackwell Publishers, 1989.

Luhtala, T.A., et al. "Dietary Restriction Attenuates Age-Related Increases in Rat Skeletal Muscle Antioxidant Enzyme Activities." *Journal of Gerontology, Biological Sciences*, Vol. 49 (1994), pp. B231–38.

Lundblad, V., and J.W. Szostak, "A Mutant with a Defect in Telomere Elongation Leads to Senescence in Yeast." *Cell*, Vol. 57 (1989), pp. 633–43.

Lustig, A.J., S. Kurtz, and D. Shore. "Involvement of the Silencer and UAS Binding Protein RAP1 in Regulation of Telomere Length." *Science*, Vol. 250 (1990), pp. 549–53.

Lytle, L.D., and A. Altar. "Diet, Central Nervous System, and Aging." *Proceedings: Federation of American Societies for Experimental Biology*, Vol. 38, No. 6 (1979), pp. 2017–22.

Malthus, Thomas R. *An Essay on the Principle of Population*. London, 1778.

——. *Population, the First Essay*. Ann Arbor, Mich.: University of Michigan Press, 1959.

Mann, D.M. "The Pathological Association Between Down Syndrome and Alzheimer's Disease." *Mechanics of Aging Development*, Vol. 43 (1993), pp. 99–36.

Marshall, E.: "NIH Picks Three Gene Vector Centers." *Science* Vol. 269 (1995), pp. 751–52.

Martin, G. "Clinical, Genetic, and Pathophysiologic Aspects of Werner's Syndrome ('Progeria of the Adult')." Paper delivered at Keystone Symposium, Molecular Biology of Aging, Lake Tahoe, 1993.

Martin, G.M., C.A. Sprague, and C.J. Epstein. "Replicative Life-span of Cultivated Human Cells: Effects of Donor's Age, Tissue and Genotype." *Laboratory Investigation*, Vol. 23 (1970), pp. 867–92.

———, et al. "Clinical, Genetic, and Pathophysiologic Aspects of Werner's Syndrome ('Progeria of the Adult')." *Journal of Cellular Biochemistry*, Supplement 17D, March 13–31, 1993. Keystone Symposium on Molecular and Cellular Biology.

Marx, J. "How a Cell Cycles Toward Cancer." *Science*, Vol. 263 (1994), pp. 319–321.

Matsuo, M. "Age-Related Alterations in Antioxidant Defense." Chapter 7 in Yu, op. cit.

McAlpine, S. (actuarial at the National Insurance Institute in New York). Personal communication, January 1995.

McClintock, B. "The Stability of Broken Ends of Chromosomes in Zea Mays." *Genetics*, Vol. 26 (1941), pp. 234–82.

Meites, J., V.W. Hylka, and W.E. Sonntag. "Need for Integration." In Roy, op. cit., pp. 187–208.

Mills, R.G., and A.S. Weiss. "Does Progeria Provide the Best Model of Accelerated Ageing in Humans?" *Gerontology*, Vol. 36 (1990), pp. 84–98.

Moore, S. *Vascular Injury and Atherosclerosis*. New York: Marcel Dekker, 1981, pp. 131–48.

Morgan, D. Personal communication, 1995.

Morin, G.B. "The Human Telomere Terminal Transferase Enzyme Is a Ribonucleoprotein That Synthesizes TTAGGG Repeats." *Cell*, Vol. 59 (1989), pp. 521–29.

Moss, N.S., and E.P. Benditt. "Human Atherosclerotic Plaque Cells and Leiomyoma Cells. Comparison of In Vitro Growth Characteristics." *American Journal of Pathology*, Vol. 78, No. 2 (1973), pp. 175–90.

Mountcastle, V.B. *Medical Physiology*, 13th ed. St. Louis: C. V. Mosby, 1974.

Moyzis, R.K. "The Human Telomere." *Scientific American*, August 1991.

Muller, H.J. "The Remaking of Chromosomes." *Collecting Net*, Vol. 13, No. 8 (1938), pp. 182–195, 198.

Nandy, K. "Effects of Antioxidant on Neuronal Lipofuscin Pigment." In Armstrong, D., et al. *Free Radiation in Molecular Biology, Aging, and Disease*. New York: Raven Press, 1984.

Nishi, R. "Neurotropic Factors: Two Are Better Than One." *Science*, Vol. 265 (1994), pp. 1052–53.

Nowak, M.A., and A.J. McMichael. "How HIV Defeats the Immune System." *Scientific American*, August 1995, pp. 58–65.

Olovnikov, A.M. [Principle of Marginotomy in Template Synthesis of Polynucleotides]. *Doklady Akademii Nauk* (SSSR), Vol. 201 (1971), pp. 1496–99.

———. "A Theory of Marginotomy: The Incomplete Copying of Template Margin in Enzymatic Synthesis of Polynucleotides and Biological Significance of the Phenomenon." *Journal of Theoretical Biology*, Vol. 41 (1973), pp. 1181–90.

Orgel, "The Maintenance of the Accuracy of Protein Synthesis and Its Relevance to Ageing," L.E. Proceedings of the National Academy of Science, Vol. 49 (1963), p. 517.

———. "Ageing Clones of Mammalian Cells." *Nature*, Vol. 243 (1973), p. 441.

———. "The Origin of Life on Earth." *Scientific American*, October 1994, pp. 77–83.

Orr, W.C., and R.S. Sohal. "Extension of Life-span by Overexpression of Superoxide Dismutase and Catalase in Drosophila Melanogaster." *Science*, Vol. 263 (1994), pp. 1128–30.

Pennisi, E. "Microglial Madness." *Science News*, Vol. 144 (1993), pp. 378–79.

Piel, G. "AIDS and Population 'Control.' " *Scientific American*, February 1994, p. 124.

Pierpaoli, W., et al. *The Melatonin Miracle*. New York: Simon & Schuster, 1995.

Pierpaoli, W., et al. *The Aging Clock: The Pineal Gland and Other Pacemakers in the Progression of Aging and Carcinogenesis. Third Stromboli Conference on Aging and Cancer.* Volume 719, Annals of the New York Academy of Science. New York: The New York Academy of Sciences, 1994.

Pimenta, W., et al. "Pancreatic Beta-Cell Dysfunction as the Primary Genetic Lesion in NIDDM." *Journal of the American Medical Association*, Vol. 273 (1995), pp. 1855–61.

Potten, C.S., and R.J. Morris. "Epithelial Stem Cells In Vivo." *Journal of Cell Science*, Supplement, Vol. 10 (1988), pp. 45–62.

Rakic, P. "DNA Synthesis and Cell Division in the Adult Primate Brain." *Annals of the New York Academy of Science*, Vol. 457 (1985), pp. 193–211.

Robbins, S.L. *Pathologic Basis of Disease*. Philadelphia: Saunders, 1974.

Rose, M.R. *Evolutionary Biology of Aging*. New York: Oxford University Press, 1991.

Ross, R. "The Pathogenesis of Atherosclerosis: An Update." *New England Journal of Medicine*, Vol. 314 (1986), pp. 488–500.

Roush, W. "Population: The View from Cairo." *Science*, Vol. 265 (1994), pp. 1164–67.

Roy, A.K., and B. Chatterjee. *Molecular Basis of Aging*. New York: Academic Press, 1984.

Ruhlen, M. *The Origin of Language*. New York: Wiley, 1994.

Samorajski, T. "How the Human Brain Responds to Aging." *Journal of the American Geriatric Society*, Vol. 24, No. 1 (1976), pp. 4–11.

Sandars, N.K., ed. *The Epic of Gilgamesh*. London: Penguin, 1960.

Sapolsky, R.M. *Stress, the Aging Brain, and Age Mechanisms of Neuron Death*. Cambridge, Mass.: MIT Press, 1992.

Sarkar, G., and M.E. Bolander. "Letters: Telomeres, Telomerase, and Cancer." *Science*, Vol. 268 (1995), pp. 1115–16.

Schmidt, A.M., et al. "Advanced Glycation Endproducts: A Mechanism for

Age-Dependent Perturbation of Monocyte and Endothelial Cell Function." *Journal of Cellular Biochemistry*, Supplement 17D, March 13–31, 1993. Keystone Symposium on Molecular and Cellular Biology.

Schneider, E.L. *Genetics of Aging*. New York: Plenum, 1978.

Seachrist, L. "Telomeres Draw a Crowd at Toronto Cancer Meeting." *Science*, Vol. 268 (1995), pp. 29–30.

———. "Hormone Mimics Fabled Fountain of Youth." *Science News*, Vol. 147 (1995), p. 391.

Sen, D. and W. Gilbert. "Novel DNA Superstructures Formed by Telomere-like Oligomers." *Biochemistry*, Vol. 31 (1992), pp. 65–70.

Service, R.F. "Dendrimers: Dream Molecules Approach Real Applications." *Science*, Vol. 267 (1995), pp. 458–59.

Singer, M., and P. Berg. *Genes and Genomes—A Changing Perspective*. Mill Valley, Calif.: University Science Books, 1991.

Skolnick, A.A. "Cancer Cells' Immortality May Prove Their Undoing." *Journal of the American Medical Association*, Vol. 273 (1995), pp. 1247–48.

Smith, D.W.E.: *Human Longevity*. New York: Oxford University Press, 1993.

Steinberg, A. "The European Colloquium on Medical Ethics: Jewish Perspectives." Given in Basel, Switzerland. Jerusalem: Magnes Press, 1989.

Stern, D. "Advanced Glycation Endproducts: A Mechanism for Age-Dependent Perturbation of Monocyte and Endothelial Cell Funtion." Paper delivered at Keystone Symposium, Molecular Biology of Aging, Lake Tahoe, 1993.

Streit, W.J., and C.A. Kincaid-Colton. "The Brain's Immune System." *Scientific American*, November 1995, pp. 54–61.

Sturrock, R.R. "Changes in Neuroglia and Myelination in the White Matter of Aging Mice." *Journal of Gerontology*, Vol. 31, No. 5 (1976), pp. 513–22.

Tan, D.X., et al. "The Pineal Hormone Melatonin Inhibits DNA-Adduct Formation Induced by the Chemical Carcinogen Safrole In Vivo." *Cancer Letters*, Vol. 70 (1993), pp. 65–71.

Terry, L.C., and J.B. Halter, "Aging of the Endocrine System." Chapter 69 in Hazzard et al., op. cit.

Tholey, G., and M. Ledig. "Plasticité neuronale et astrocytaire: aspects metaboliques" ("Neuronal and Astrocytic Plasticity: Metabolic Aspects"). Annales de Medecine Interne (Paris), Vol. 141, Suppl. 1 (1990), pp. 13–18.

Thorn, G.W., et al. *Harrison's Principles of Internal Medicine*, 8th Ed. New York: McGraw-Hill, 1977.

Travis, J. "Glia: The Brain's Other Cells." *Science*, Vol. 266 (1995), pp. 970–72.

Vaziri H; et al. "Loss of Telomeric DNA During Aging of Normal and Trisomy 21 Human Lymphocytes." *American Journal of Human Genetics*, Vol. 52 (1993), p. 661.

———, et al. "Evidence for a Mitotic Clock in Human Hematopoietic Stem Cells: Loss of Telomeric DNA with Age." *Proceedings of the National Academy of Science*, Vol. 91, October 11, 1994.

Vernadakis, A. "Neuronal-Glial Interactions During Development and Aging." *Fed. Proc.*, Vol. 34, No. 1 (1975), pp. 89–95.

Voelker, R. "Ames Agrees with Mom's Advice: Eat Your Fruits and Vegetables." *Journal of the American Medical Association*, Vol. 273 (1995), pp. 1077–78.

Walters, L. *Journal of Clinical Ethics*, Vol. 2 (1991), p. 267.

Watson, J.D. *The Double Helix*. New York: Mentor, 1968.

———. "Origin of Concatameric T7 DNA." *Nature: New Biology*, Vol. 239 (1972), pp. 197–201.

Wei, X., et al. "Viral Dynamics in Human Immunodeficiency Virus Type 1 Injection." *Nature*, Vol. 373 (1995), p. 117.

Weindruch, R., H.R. Warner, and P.E. Starke-Reed. "Future Directions of Free Radical Research in Aging." Chapter 12 in Yu, op. cit.

Weiner, A.M. "Eukaryotic Nuclear Telomeres: Molecular Fossils of the RNP World?" *Cell*, Vol. 52 (1988), pp. 155–57.

Weir, G.C. "Which Comes First in Non-Insulin-Dependent Diabetes Mellitus: Insulin Resistance or Beta-Cell Failure? Both Come First." *Journal of the American Medical Association*, Vol. 273 (1995), pp. 1878–79.

Wise, P.M., et al. "Neuroendocrine Concomitants of Reproductive Aging." *Experimental Gerontology*, Vol. 29 (1994), pp. 275–84.

Wivel, N.A., and L. Walters. "Germ-line Modification and Disease Prevention: Some Medical and Ethical Perspectives." *Science*, Vol. 262 (1993), pp. 533–38.

World Almanac, 1992.

Wright, W.E., and J.W. Shay. "Re-expression of Senescent Markers in Deinduced Reversibly Immortalized Cells." *Experimental Gerontology*, Vol. 27, No. 5–6 (1992), pp. 477–92.

———, and J.W. Shay. "Telomere Positional Effects and the Regulation of Cellular Senescence." *Trends in Genetics*, Vol. 8 (1992), pp. 193–97.

Yu, B.P. *Free Radicals in Aging*. Boca Raton, Fla.: CRC Press, 1993.

Yu, G.L., and E.H. Blackburn. "Amplification of Tandemly Repeated Origin Control Sequences Confers a Replication Advantage on rDNA Replicons in Tetrahymena Thermophila." *Mol. Cell. Biol.*, Vol. 10, No. 5 (1990), pp. 2070–80.

———, et al. "In Vivo Alteration of Telomere Sequences and Senescence Caused by Mutated Tetrahymena Telomerase RNAs." *Nature*, Vol. 344, No. 6262 (1990), pp. 126–32.

Zakian, V.A. "Structure and Function of Telomeres." *Annual Review of Genetics*, Vol. 23 (1989), pp. 579–604.

Zayn al-' Abidin, A. *Sahifa al-Sajjadiyya*, trans. William Chittick. London: Oxford University Press, 1988.

INDEX